1. Missions. Korea. 2. Korea.

I. Title.

The Quality of Mercy

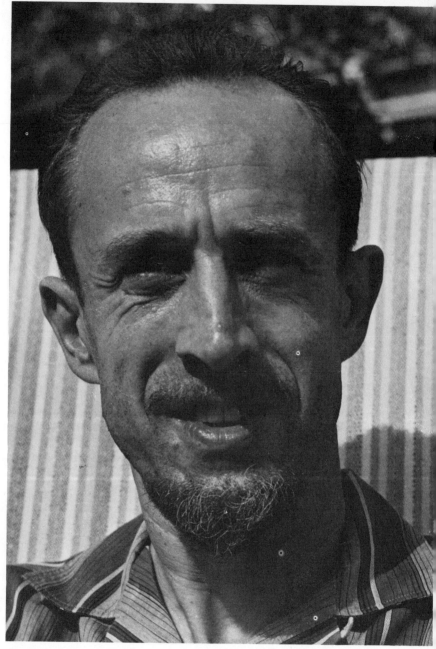

John Steensma.

Photo by Pak, Yo-il Leika Studio, Taejon

The
Quality
of Mercy

by Juliana Steensma

 JOHN KNOX PRESS
Richmond, Virginia

Standard Book Number: 8042-1496-4
Library of Congress Catalog Card Number: 69-13271
© M. E. Bratcher 1969
Printed in the United States of America

HV
1559
, K8
573

To "Sir" with Love

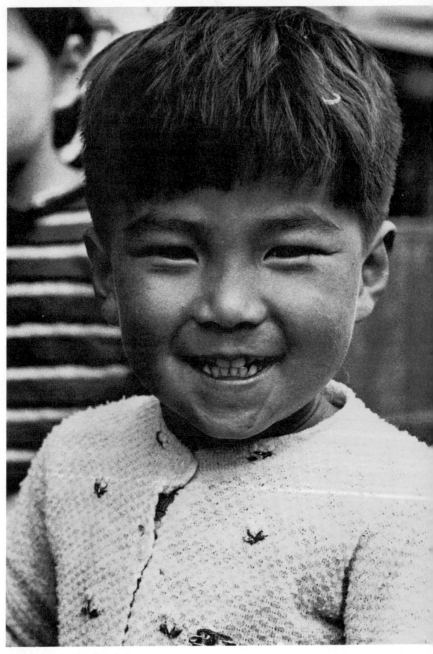
Happiness is Korea's future.

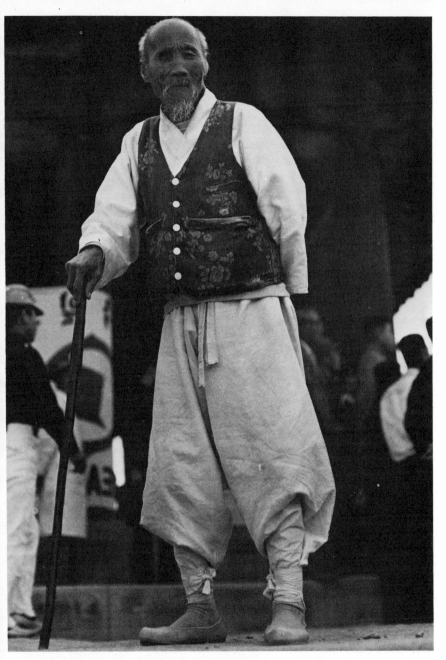

Happiness is the heritage of Korea's ancient culture.
Photos by Robert Ebert, Honolulu

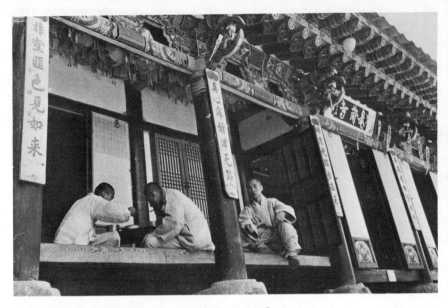

Buddhist monks enjoy supper on their front porch.

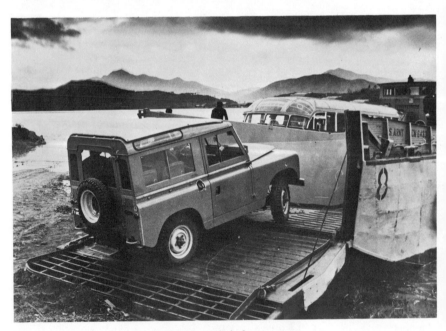

There are places even a Land Rover needs help to get to.
Photos by Robert Ebert, Honolulu

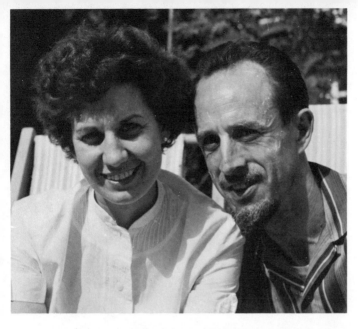

John
and
Juliana
Steensma.

*Photo by
Pak, Yo-il
Leika Studio,
Taejon*

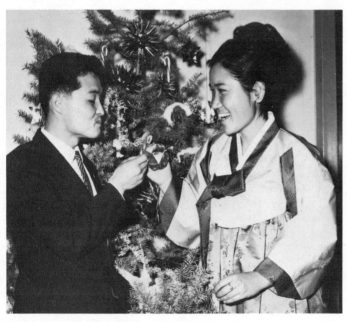

Mr. Chun
and
Miss Koh.

Their romance points the way to the future.

The
Quality
of Mercy

1

The young man who stood on my doorstep had a problem. That was not hard to see. After eight years of living in Korea, we were accustomed to finding people with problems in front of our door. We were American Christians who had come to Korea with the professed intention of helping Korean people, and American missionaries who preach the love and mercy of Jesus Christ are fair game for those who make their living by begging from door to door. We were very much aware of our Lord's words, "Verily I say unto you, Inasmuch as ye did it not to one of the least of these, ye did it not to me" (Matt. 25:45, K.J.V.).

Their stories were all alike. The beggars who came to our door were all orphans and refugees, all widowed or sick. And the only kind of help they ever wanted was a handout.

Mr. Chun was obviously different. Handsome and well-dressed, he immediately charmed me with his apologetic greeting and an embarrassed smile.

"I need your advice," he said. "Will you help me with your experience?"

There is nothing which pleases a woman of my age more than to be asked for advice, especially on problems of love. This seemed to be the area of Mr. Chun's difficulty and when he told me about it I could understand his problem immediately.

"I have love for Miss Koh," he stated simply. We both knew that this was not a simple problem, for Miss Koh was a double leg amputee. My thoughts slipped back twenty years to the time when I admitted to myself that there was only one man who would do as my husband. This should have been a happy decision; instead it was a time of agonizing uncertainty.

John Steensma had all the qualifications for a good husband— he was intelligent and friendly, he seemed responsible, and we shared the same faith. I was attracted by the mischief in his eyes and encouraged by his genuine commitment to the ideals which formed the core of my own life. Physically he was not unattractive, better looking than average, neat, and conservative in dress.

Yet my friends made excuses when we asked them to go out with us in public and they admitted to me privately that, although my fiance was a good-enough fellow, it made them "feel funny" to be with him. Teachers, preachers, and other voluntary counselors took me aside and advised me with the best of intentions to terminate the romance. I was young, and perhaps I did not realize that a union such as we contemplated was a mistake. The man whom I had chosen simply was not a good risk.

This was obvious to everyone but me. I knew John. Others saw only that he had lost both arms and they could not see beyond this. They were blind to the courage, determination, and stability of character that made this young man different and outstanding.

Until the end of his seventeenth year, John's life had been very normal. He had been raised in a family of eight children by hard-working immigrant parents who communicated their strong faith in God to their children. Home was a warm and secure place where everyone felt loved and wanted and enjoyed a boisterous companionship in work and play. Times were not easy; it was difficult for the father to earn a living for this large family. But Mother Steensma was a shrewd manager and she taught her children never to borrow worry from tomorrow. All shared the responsibilities of the busy household; all money earned outside was contributed to the family pot; family loyalty and solidarity were taken for granted.

The parents did not encourage their children to pursue education beyond elementary school, and only John showed any desire to do so. His desire to go to school was probably motivated less by love of learning than by the opportunity to drive a rattling

"Model T" three miles across the city twice a day. Perhaps it was a preference for baseball practice with the high school team to a day of hard work with his brothers on Pa's truck that made John stay in school. At any rate, the name of John Steensma appeared on the roll of graduates from the Christian High School in Grand Rapids, Michigan, in the summer of 1939.

If John had been asked that summer about his plans for the future, he might have laughed. He was enjoying himself, living each day with the exuberance and thoughtlessness of youth. He drove his father's truck as it collected loads of sawdust and shavings from the furniture factories in Grand Rapids and he helped his brothers in the mill as they ground it up, bagged it, and delivered it to meat markets and other customers who had use for it. This business not only kept the five young Steensma boys busy, but it also supported a family of relatives. The cousins were all boys of the same age, so that the work often turned into horseplay as the feisty young men jostled and wrestled each other in the warehouse.

So it was on that rainy day in October of 1939 when for John Steensma life suddenly changed direction. No one felt much like working and soon the younger boys abandoned even the pretense. One of them suggested making a parachute out of the burlap bags.

"We could float it down off that tower there," he said.

It sounded like an interesting idea, and when Abie, who was the eldest, stopped tying his sacks of sawdust and tossed his ball of twine over to the parachute-makers, the vote to quit working was unanimous. The whole gang of cousins scrambled up the electric tower, paying no heed to the large letters on the sign at the bottom:

"DANGER! 72,000 VOLTS!"

Someone threw the parachute from the top of the tower. Halfway down the wind caught it and it stuck there, draped over the wires. Two or three of the boys began to scramble nimbly toward it, but John was quicker than any of them. Hands grasping the arm of the steel framework, he swung out like a monkey and kicked at the piece of burlap which hung on the wire beneath. This is the last he remembers.

The others tell about the ball of fire, the shrill scream, the limp body dropping the long seventy-five feet to the ground. The high-tension current had drawn the boy's foot to it, passed through his body, and grounded itself on the steel bar which he had held in his hands. The doctors thought that the electric charge had killed him; but the heart which stopped beating was shocked back into action when the unconscious body hit the ground. Although he was breathing when he entered the hospital, no one expected him to live through the night.

In the haze of semiconsciousness, John listened to the discussions of the doctors around his bed, and he made up his mind that he would *not* die. He heard his mother's moan of agony when she was told that both his hands were burned away. He played the game bravely when nurses and visitors tried to hide from him the loss of his hands, and he bore his suffering without complaint. Yet he was acutely aware of the change in his circumstances. Resolutely keeping his thoughts from the future, he concentrated upon getting well.

There were days of despair, when the torture of the burned body drove everything else from his mind. There were even days when he longed to die—when the struggle for life seemed too much for his strength. The day the surgeon came in and told him very, very gently that gangrene had set in at the elbow and the right arm would have to be reamputated near the shoulder was such a day. The boy cried then . . . because he was barely eighteen and because he wanted to play baseball again.

There were days of victory too, as each succeeding crisis passed and the patient took another step toward recovery. One day followed another, and John took them one at a time. In that process, the boy became a man.

When I met him, three years afterward, he had learned to use the clumsy artificial arms with skill. America was at war then, and John had found a job in a defense plant. Every man was needed, and those who were not physically fit for military service took their places in the factories at home.

All of this was a long time ago. We are both older and wiser now, and it is so easy to look back upon the past and see the path which has led up to the present. We can see the turnings which have changed the direction of our lives and we can evaluate the influences which resulted in the decisions we made. For my husband, it was clear enough. When he lost his hands, he was forced to come to a standstill and to take stock of himself. He realized that his life had been aimless and pleasant, and he could see that that phase of it had come to an end.

We never meant to fall in love. I was a college student, interested in social work. Impressed by John's determination to be independent, I went out of my way to help him. Education seemed a sensible course to follow, and so John enrolled at Calvin College in Grand Rapids, where I was already in my third year. Soon we were doing most of our studying together as he tried to overcome the handicaps of poor academic preparation, a four-year gap between high school and college, and a physical disability that made note-taking difficult and writing on the blackboard impossible. The teamwork was effective. John used my hands when he needed them, and I leaned upon his organizational abilities to make better use of my time. People shook their heads when John told them he wanted to become a foreign missionary—they had never heard of a missionary without hands. My father became very distressed when we wrote him of our plan to marry.

He replied: "Have you reasonable assurance that there are no material difficulties? If John is studying he can earn no money and times are likely to change for the worse. Your parents are not wealthy, nor are his and we cannot help you. Have you considered all this? Remember that John will have to study for several years yet and then, when he reaches a goal things are still uncertain. Of course, it is well to have confidence in a person and to trust that the Lord will provide, but Scripture teaches us also to estimate the cost of a tower before we build it, lest we are unable to finish it. I do not wish to throw cold water on your enthusiasm, but it is my solemn duty to do so. Please face your future as it should be faced."

Hardly an encouragement!

My heart reached out in understanding to Mr. Chun, for I knew the obstacles he would face if he wanted to marry the lovely

Miss Koh. America has changed a great deal since the day I decided to face prejudice with John Steensma. Returning war amputees and a program of public education have gradually altered the attitude of people toward the disabled. When given a chance, those who had been crippled by birth or by accident have proved beyond a doubt that they could compete with normal individuals and they were soon accepted by the same standards. Progress in prosthetics and in rehabilitation techniques helped, but the big jump forward was the shift in public thinking.

In Korea there has been progress too, since those days when the disabled were hidden from the eyes of the public or chased out of the family to beg. Still, there remains enough of the old superstition, the old prejudice, and the old pride so that the average parent would not welcome a crippled daughter-in-law. Mr. Chun knew this very well and he realized that I knew it also. Although he summed up the whole problem in a few words, we were both aware of its far-reaching implications.

"I love Miss Koh," repeated Mr. Chun. "But how can we marry?"

2

Chun Bong Yoon was the youngest and the handsomest of the social caseworkers at the Korea Church World Service Amputee Rehabilitation Center in Seoul. He had graduated from the Seoul National University and had come to the Center with excellent recommendations. The problems of the disabled were his special interest, and his earnestness and sincerity communicated itself as he counseled the handicapped that they must learn to believe in themselves if they expected to be accepted by others.

He was assisted in his work by our latest addition to the staff, the beautiful and vivacious Miss Koh. She soon won his regard by her efficient manner and by her complete self-sufficiency. This was no shrinking Korean maiden who giggled behind a fan, but a modern, educated young woman who knew the direction she wanted to go. She asked no favors, but went about her work with a competence and a good nature that won the affection of all who met her. Often as visitors were guided around the rehabilitation center by Miss Koh, they were so charmed by her flashing eyes and dimpled smile that they failed to notice that she walked on two artificial legs. The patients with whom she played Ping-Pong were kept so busy by her wicked return of the ball that they had no time to wonder at her fast footwork. At basketball she was an asset to her team, and on weekends she went mountain climbing with her boyfriends. Nothing stopped Miss Koh, and those of us who worked with her had long ago become unconscious of any disability. We accepted her artificial legs as casually as she herself had accepted them.

When Koh Yung Sook first came to the Center, she discovered a whole new world. Her parents, with love and understanding, had taught her to accept responsibility, even though she was crippled. At the amputee center she saw children who had been rejected and abandoned because they were amputees. She talked to fathers who were unable to provide a living for their families. She met young people who had no hope in life and who were willing to give up without really trying. All of this appalled her. She volunteered to serve as an assistant to the social workers, and her services were gladly accepted. Her bright cheeriness became an encouragement to patients and staff members alike and she was easily the most popular member of the entire group. Mr. Chun had taken a special liking to this promising assistant, and he was intensely interested in her adjustment to her handicap. He spent much time with her, advising her and consulting her, and discussing with her how it was possible for an amputee to live a full and useful life.

Gradually these conferences took on added meaning, as the two young people began to understand each other's point of view. They shared their knowledge and they shared a concern for the people with whom they were working. They shared their ideas and their hopes and their dreams; and as we watched, they began to share their love for each other. We wondered then what would happen, as we remembered the time of our own youth.

Mr. Chun played it softly as long as he could. Affairs came to a climax when Miss Koh's father announced that he planned to emigrate to Brazil and take his family with him. Unless he decided very quickly to marry Miss Koh, Mr. Chun faced almost certain separation from the girl he confessed that he loved.

He had not told his family about it. He knew already what their reaction would be. They had never met an amputee and they would be shocked and dismayed by his choice. As refugees from North Korea, they had suffered hardship and want and had made great sacrifices in order that this youngest son might have a good education and make an acceptable marriage. Their hopes were fixed on him and he knew it.

"Try to see it their way," he had pleaded with Miss Koh. And she *had* tried. Out of her love for him, out of her years of experience as a handicapped girl in a world full of normal people, she had tried to see herself as she must look to them.

Mr. Chun felt helpless. He was a dutiful son, but he loved Miss Koh so much that he could not face the prospect of losing her. The day of departure for Brazil came closer. Mr. Chun became desperate. He must make a decision.

I told him about my own father.

"It is not easy," I said, "but often it becomes better. Perhaps together you and Miss Koh can pioneer the way for other amputees in Korea so that after another twenty years no one will have this problem anymore."

Mr. Chun smiled at me. "Miss Koh is very wonderful," he said in his precisely articulated English. "When you and Mr. Steensma return to America, we must become the leaders for the disabled Korean people."

And so, a few months later, we were invited to their wedding. As we watched the lovely bride walk with a sure and certain step toward her bridegroom, we wished them well with overflowing hearts. They were so confident and they were so young. They loved each other and they loved their own people. They knew that they would meet with prejudice and with misunderstanding, but they accepted the role of pioneers. Together they wished to fight the barriers of bigotry and discrimination that are a hangover from the old Korea. We cannot believe that they will fail.

It was time for us to leave Korea—to leave the work with the handicapped in the hands of people like Mr. and Mrs. Chun. During the eight years that we lived and worked in Korea we carefully planned for this time of leaving. Gradually and deliberately we had turned over responsibilities to trained Korean staff members and we had tried to teach them our skills and the lessons of our experience. By word and by example we had also tried to leave our ideals with them and to impress them with the conviction that surrender to Christ includes service to our neighbor.

Korea has been very good to us and Korea has been good for

us. It was not easy to break the ties of love which bound us to this country and its people. But Korean people have demonstrated that they are capable and ready to assume leadership and to take care of themselves. When we returned to the churches which had sent us, we could assure them that if the Korean people are given the same cooperation, assistance, and consideration which was given to us as foreigners, they can do the same job as well or better than we have done it.

That may be hard for some Americans to accept. Most of us enjoy the paternalistic relationship which missionaries often establish in a foreign country, especially in those places which have suffered the effects of war, deprivation, or isolation. We often seek to preserve our image as the Lord's special ambassadors. We forget that, as foreigners, we have no right to stay longer than we are needed in a country where there is not enough room for the native citizens and where some of them might possibly be able to perform the jobs which we have been sent to accomplish.

The Church World Service Amputee Rehabilitation Center had now become established as a part of the Yonsei University Medical Complex. It had earned a reputation in the three years of its existence as the outstanding limb manufacturer in the country. Students of social work from four of the leading Korean universities vied for the opportunity to take their fieldwork training at the Christian rehabilitation center. Doctors from the large national and mission medical centers sent their patients to the Church World Service Center for rehabilitation. The Shrine Club, a group of Americans who sponsor crippled children, was supporting a social worker on the staff of the Center to work with the children who were being helped by the money raised by the club members. Another social worker went out to minister to leprosy patients, visiting them in the leprosy colonies and seeking to prepare their homes and villages to receive them after they had been healed and rehabilitated. This outreach was supported by a grant from the American Leprosy Mission. A part-time chaplain-counselor and a chapel ministry was made possible as a part of the work of rehabilitation by gifts sent to us by friends in our own home church.

Most encouraging of all, several of the staff members decided on their own to begin a voluntary program to promote the welfare of all Koreans who are physically handicapped in one way or another. Their aim was to reduce prejudice and to create understanding between the handicapped and the non-handicapped. The effort began with public education and with the publication of a small monthly magazine containing the stories of those who had overcome their disabilities, and also advice and encouragement to those who were depressed by handicaps.

There were many obstacles and much frustration before the first issue of this little magazine was ready for distribution. The Korean government has strict regulations on publication, and piles of papers had to be filled out and filed with the various government offices. Weeks of negotiation and months of waiting passed before the approval to publish "The Rehabilitated" was granted. Two thousand copies of the first issue were sent out. More than half the people to whom it was sent had not subscribed for it, but within the first month seven hundred Korean people sent in subscriptions. To appreciate this enthusiastic response, one must look back to the beginnings of the work in amputee rehabilitation in Korea. One must remember the dark, difficult days in 1951 when the pitiful, maimed victims of the Korean War were turned out on the streets because there was no room for them in the hospitals. When a Korean hospital superintendent begged an American missionary to present the problem of these maimed outcasts to the Christian churches in America, relief was quick to come.

To Dr. Reuben A. Torrey, Jr., who responded to that plea and came to Korea in 1952 to work with Korean amputees, the dedication of this group of Korean rehabilitation workers to the acceptance of the disabled in Korean society was the culmination of years of prayer, hard work, and sacrifice. After serving as a missionary in China for many years, Dr. Torrey had lost his right arm in an accident. Forced out of China by the Communist takeover and retired from mission service by the loss of his arm, Dr. Torrey was quick to see the call to Korea as a unique opportunity to demonstrate by his own example that amputees can live normal lives and be of service to others.

The first need was for artificial limbs for the hundreds of am-

putees who came seeking help. With the loss of an arm or a leg these
people had lost all human dignity. In a desperate economy where
there was not enough food for a whole man, the cripple was pushed
out. In the city of Taejon, located at the geographical center of
Korea, Dr. Torrey established a vocational training center for amputees. The aim of the Center was to restore to these beaten cripples their self-respect by making them productive citizens again.
Women learned weaving and knitting, embroidery and sewing. The
men were taught animal husbandry, carpentry, bamboo work, metal
shop, machine shop, and tailoring. Child amputees were enrolled
in local schools under the sponsorship of the Oxford Famine Relief
Committee of England and other overseas relief organizations. The
emphasis and atmosphere at the Center were Christian and mutual
helpfulness was stressed. Gradually the little community developed
in its beautiful natural setting. Amputees were given jobs on the
staff as maintenance workers, instructors in the various shops, office
assistants, limb makers. They lived in houses on the Center grounds
and their children played with the amputee children from the dormitories. A resident evangelist conducted services in the chapel,
supervised the Sunday school and midweek meetings, and was
responsible for the spiritual welfare of all the members of the Center
settlement.

For seven years Dr. Torrey carried on this tireless effort to
restore as many amputees as he possibly could reach in Korea. He
traveled up and down the country from Pusan to Seoul, by rail and
by jeep. He spent hours in his poorly-heated little office, laboriously
working his way through budgets and accounts, reports and case
histories, writing letters to donors, to churches, and to friends. Yet
he was always ready to listen when people came to ask him for help.
To the people of Korea he became known as "the grandfather who
loves us" and as such he will always be remembered.

Dr. Torrey gave his heart to the amputees of Korea, but he was
seventy-one years old and his strength began to fail. It was time
for a rest and he had to look for a replacement. Was there a man,
anywhere, who was trained in rehabilitation, experienced in prosthetics, interested in missionary service? Dr. Torrey did not dare
to hope. Instead, he prayed. He trusted God to locate the man who

could take over his job and continue the work of rehabilitation which he had begun in Korea.

He did not know that God had already prepared a man for that very task.

3

M y memories of our first few weeks in Korea in the autumn
of 1958 are a bittersweet mixture of discovery and appre-
hension. Like most Americans, we had seen pictures and
heard stories of appalling conditions in Korea, of starving orphans
and abandoned children, of slums and shacks, dirt and depression.
I do not remember anything good that was said about this little
country, and naturally I did not look forward to an easy life there.
But I was determined to love Korea.

As it turned out, this was the easiest part of the entire experience. The beautiful Korean autumn and the warm welcome given
to us by the Korean people won us over completely within a few
days after arrival. On the first Sunday we were given a formal
welcome at the chapel service of the amputee center. After the
service the evangelist spoke to the people and to us, and all responded with upraised hands and wide smiles. Then one young man
volunteered to sing a solo as a special welcome. He sang in Korean
to the tune of "Jesus Wants Me for a Sunbeam" and although we
could not understand his words, we appreciated the beauty of his
voice and his effort to sing something that would sound familiar
to our children.

The service that first Sunday was an inspiration for us. We had
been told that many of the amputees who came there heard of
Christ for the first time. As we sat among the halt and the maimed
we were struck by the devotion and the real spirit of worship which

24

they showed. During the service, twenty-one young amputees were accepted as candidates for baptism. They came to the front of the gathering, supporting each other and leaning on their crutches and canes. They were accepted into the church as "learners" and would spend the next six months on a sort of probation, during which time they would be counseled, taught in Scripture, and encouraged in Christian conduct. After that they could be baptized. Thirteen adults received the sacrament of baptism that day and four children of parents who had already become Christians were baptized at the same service. Most of these people had had their first contact with Christianity at the amputee center.

The service was very long, and when I returned to our house the dinner which had been cooking in the oven was a scorched mess. No one had explained the water pump to us, so when it shut itself off automatically we were without water for the rest of the day. The children had no toys, no playmates, and no experience in entertaining themselves, so they soon became cross and complained. During the first few weeks we lived with the bare necessities, which we had borrowed from other missionaries. The electric power went off each evening for several hours and we wrote letters by candlelight. We had no radio and no books so we usually went to bed around nine o'clock. Although this is a Korean way of life, it was a new way for an American family fresh from a city in the United States.

Going to bed was not a peaceful experience either. Thoughtful "friends" had briefed us on the habits of the notorious Korean "slickee boys" and the idea of strangers sneaking into our bedrooms to steal was terrifying for me. I lay awake, straining at the slightest sounds and trembling when the dogs began to bark. Although I heard no thieves, the patter of the rats in the walls behind the headboard was disturbing enough. They sounded so close that two or three times in the night I had to put on the light to assure myself that they were not in the room with me. My skin itched and crawled, with nervousness—I thought. It was not until we had lived in the house for two weeks that I found the fleas in our bed and identified the little red bites on my body.

There were other problems. Several of our Methodist, Southern Presbyterian, and Southern Baptist missionary neighbors had started a school for their children. The mothers taught them in a little Quonset hut, using the Calvert correspondence courses. Mary, our youngest, was put into the kindergarten taught by a young Korean woman. She hated it from the first. "All those kids can talk Korean but me," she complained.

She also hated the walk across the rice paddies from our house to the school. We had to use steppingstones to get across the creek and invariably, Mary stepped into the cold water. I tried to get her across by carrying her on my back, but eventually decided that it was easier to take off the children's shoes and stockings and let them wade through. As soon as we hit upon this solution we were warned by more experienced missionaries of the danger of hookworm in the Korean mud.

Joy, who was six, was happy in the first grade. There was another little girl of the same age and the two became friends at once. But Dirk found no children his age, with the exception of one Baptist girl. At ten years of age boys hate girls more than anything else in the world. Every day, Dirk and I trudged over to the Quonset school and I tried to teach him the Calvert material for the fifth grade. He made no effort to conceal his boredom. I was his mother, and he would not accept me as his teacher.

As for the oldest child, a girl of twelve, we had neither study materials nor a teacher for her. Nor was there anyone near her age for her to talk to or play with. She had strenuously objected to the move to Korea and her isolation and inactivity did not make her any easier to live with now that we had arrived. Altogether, it was very discouraging.

We had no idea what sort of food was available on the Korean market, and our innocence of Korean language did not make the purchasing any easier. When I was confronted with the open-air stall where the meat was covered with flies and handled by all the customers, it no longer seemed desirable to eat meat. And when I had to elbow my way through the curious crowds and submit to their stares and comments I usually lost my courage before I had managed to buy anything. Our cook was helpful, but she knew not a word of English. She gave us her sympathy and she did her best, but those first few weeks were awful.

When I had reached the apex of homesickness, loneliness, nervousness, and frustration, deliverance arrived in a suggestion of the Korea Church World Service Director that we move to Seoul. There we could spend a few months attending Korean language school while our children were enrolled in the Seoul Foreign School for missionary children. It was exactly the right solution. Living in Seoul gave us the chance to adjust gradually to the life in Korea. At language school we met other new missionaries and we compared notes and encouraged each other. When the drains froze or the city water was shut off for three days, we knew where to go for help. We could call the Church World Service offices whenever we became desperate and so we no longer had to carry the whole burden of responsibility for the family which we had brought to this strange, foreign country.

The old Japanese house which we occupied in Seoul was pleasant and interesting, although it became too cold in the winter. Each room was heated by its own oil stove, and sometimes the temperature dropped so far that the oil became too thick to move through the pipe and then the stove went out. We were walled in, with a big front gate and a small gate in the rear. When friends came to call, they would sound the car horn or call out to us over the wall. There was also an electric buzzer which sounded inside the house. It made us feel very elegant, and it also gave us a sense of protection. A little gate inside the main gate led into a lovely Japanese garden with flowers and a stone lantern beside a lily pond. Underneath it all was an old bomb shelter which the children found exciting to explore.

Before long the Korean children in the neighborhood realized that a family of Americans had moved in behind the wall. They often stood on each other's hands outside and peeked over the stone wall to watch our children at play. Then they would practice the meager English that they learned at school and call out to us, "I am Korean school-boy. Boy-friend, will you play-ball with me?" Once a Korean schoolboy tossed his peaked cap into the garden and our little girls seized upon it as a new toy. We remembered that day a week later as we soaked their long hair with kerosene and picked out the nits of the lice which had come along with the cap.

A night guard was hired to patrol the place all night, but it was a long time before I was able to overcome the night jitters. Before we went to bed we put a padlock on the outside gate, bolted all the doors, and hid all our possessions such as cameras, radio, overcoats, in a closet with a lock. Often during the night I would awaken and lie for hours listening for the steps of the guard. I learned to listen for the clack-clack of the sticks with which the neighborhood watchman informed us of his passing. Late at night and before dawn the street peddlers cried out their wares. As I learned to know the sounds, they became a reassuring lullaby, a background music for our night's rest.

The daily drive to language school gave us an opportunity to become familiar with the city. We were amazed by the number of jeep-type vehicles we saw in the streets, but it did not take much imagination to figure out why after we had traveled over the bumpy roads ourselves. The jeeps came in all sizes and colors and the fancier ones were equipped with ruffled curtains at the windows. It seemed to us that they behaved oddly too—there were no traffic regulations as far as we could tell. In order to avoid the holes in the streets, avoid the people who walked in groups of three or four or more and paid no attention to the vehicles, avoid the bicycles with their huge loads and the push carts and animals which filled the roads, the cars drove in and out from one side to the other.

Our children were amused by the sight of the Korean men who walked from the public bath to their homes in pajamas. And I was also astonished the first time I rode on the train to see a gentleman rise from his seat, remove his coat and necktie and shirt, and then proceed to take off his trousers. He carefully hung up all his outer clothing and settled down comfortably in his pajamas. Certainly, it was a sensible thing to do. When he approached his destination he donned his clothes again and stepped off the train without spot or wrinkle.

Every day brought new excitement. One never knew what might happen next. One Sunday, after the afternoon church service, we were greeting one another in the lobby. Suddenly a man fell from above and landed at our feet. He had been in the gallery and the section of floor under him had unexpectedly given way. So he came through the ceiling above our heads. The young man picked himself up, brushed the plaster dust off his suit, and walked away as if such a thing happened to him every day.

On another Sunday, John was invited to speak to a group of refugees, many of whom were amputees. We found the church in the middle of a tent camp where a large group of people maintained a precarious struggle for existence. The conditions in that camp furnished the raw material for the tear-jerking stories which had made Korea's reputation. Infants played naked in the dust on the pathways, while older brothers and sisters kept an eye on them. Old men sat in groups, playing chess games on the ground with stones. The women were busy carrying water, cooking, and washing out the clothing. A large following was quickly attracted by the foreign visitors who made their way through the alleyways to the crude church building.

A crowd of ragged people already packed the inside of the church. The ladies sat nursing their babies on the floor at the speaker's left. On the other side of the aisle were the men and boys. In the rear, at the door, stood the custodian of the shoes. We filed our footwear away on the shelf with the rubber shoes of the others and were led away to a guest bench and seated on a cushion next to the platform.

With the aid of an interpreter, John told the people how God had led him and prepared him through all his life for this task in Korea. He described the work which was being done in the name of Christ and the joy and hope which we had seen among the Christian amputees in the Taejon center. The people listened with attention. Those who could not find a place inside hung in the open windows. After the meeting had ended, we were deeply moved by the appreciation shown by the audience. We lingered to greet old grandmothers whose tears fell on my hands as they kissed them, young men who crawled toward us on their stumped legs, a row of young women amputees who sat on a bench by the door, and a multitude of dirty, friendly little children who followed us all the way to the road where we caught our bus for home.

The pastor who brought us to this group told us that he had

a list of three hundred amputees who lived in the city of Seoul—
people who had received no artificial limbs and no help. We began
to wonder how we could find room for all those people in the
already overcrowded amputee center at Taejon. There was no question of the need. It was up to us to find some way to offer help to
all the amputees in Korea.

4

The friends in Taejon had predicted that once people grow accustomed to the fast social pace in the capital city, they do not want to return to the country to live. Seoul certainly was an exciting city. There was a good-sized international colony and the headquarters of the U.S. forces were all in Seoul also. Something was always happening.

Our home soon became a "home away from home" for American servicemen whom we met at the chapel, which we attended, or who were referred to us by the committee on servicemen of the churches back home. These fellows became regular visitors; it was a rare Sunday that we dined alone. Sometimes they stayed overnight, or for the weekend. More often they would drop in unexpectedly, bringing with them goodies from the PX to add to the meal. We reciprocated by introducing them to the sights and sounds of Seoul and taking them on tours to points of interest.

Language school was not easy. Neither of us had been in school for many, many years and our brains seemed to have rusted. The method used was that of memorizing sentences from a book which had been written many years before by a veteran American missionary. Each day's lesson presented a different verb form. One day the class had to learn how to say "can do"; the next, "must do"; and then, "am going to do," "allow to do," and on and on. I learned a great deal in that language school, but I did not learn to speak Korean. It seemed that the method of teaching was upside down, and although the teacher agreed with that opinion, he was paid to teach the material that he had been given to teach. So every day he struggled to teach a new grammatical construction while the students forgot what they had learned on the day before. Since we did not learn root verbs, we could not use the words except in the sentences that had been memorized. The theory was that if one learned the pattern sentences well, they would become second nature and one could use them naturally in conversation. But what can you do with a sentence pattern like this: "Even though I die, I will not betray my Lord"? There was no use for it with the cook or the driver or the laundress—or anyone else, so it was quickly forgotten.

One of the sentences was so silly that I never forgot it. I learned to say in Korean language, "Are you going to commit suicide?" but it was not a useful sentence. When I tried it out on the night guard he was greatly amused and he told me about the signs which could be found on the cliffs which bordered the Han River near Seoul City. Spring in Korea brings out all the melancholy feelings which have been stored up throughout the winter, he explained to me. People begin to brood upon unhappy love affairs in the past and they remember sins which have caused unhappiness to themselves or to others. So many try to kill themselves by leaping into the Han that the police finally posted a sign by the river: "If you jump you will be prosecuted!"

"I think," observed our Mr. Kim wryly, "every spring the prison must be full of suicides."

Our children loved their new school, and this immediately made life much more pleasant for the entire family. The companionship of children from all of the different missions and from every part of the United States, from Sweden, Turkey, Britain, Australia, Japan, Korea, Germany, France, Thailand, and Italy was stimulating and different. Seoul Foreign School was international, but the education was American, conforming to the standards of the states of New York and California. The children learned the different sports of other countries and soon learned to be world citizens.

Mary started school in a kindergarten run by the wife of an American aid representative. We were able to learn a great deal about the conditions of rural Korea from her husband during that year.

Little Mary made friends easily. She was a bundle of energy, pretty and vivacious. The Korean people found her captivating, with her cottony white hair and her sparkling eyes and friendly manner. Joy, in contrast, was quiet and uncomplicated and easy to have around. Although she is the younger of the two, Mary always took the lead in new situations and Joy depended upon her for support. One morning Mary announced to us that she intended to pay a call on our Korean neighbors. She dressed up in her holiday costume (a gift from our employees on our first Christmas in Korea), spent fifteen minutes with a cup of water on her hair, and marched next door to visit. The members of the family next door were important people in Seoul. They had all studied in America and were prominent figures in civic and international organizations.

Mary was admitted, made a curtsy, and greeted her hostess in Korean language. She stayed for more than two hours, while we all wondered what a Korean matron and a garrulous five-year-old American child could find to talk about. But when Mary returned she was disgusted. Yes, the lady was nice—but she talked "all English" and Mary was very proud of the little bit of Korean language she had learned in kindergarten.

During this first year of adjustment we saw many new sights and learned many new things. We saw our first "demo" when the people protested Japan's decision to send Koreans back to North Korea. Children left their schoolrooms and marched in the streets, carrying placards. We knew that the hatred between Korea and Japan was deep and long-standing but we could not see what the political demonstration would accomplish. But we learned that demonstrations are a part of life in the Orient and that the participants could become very nasty and uncontrolled.

We learned new habits. One was not to push on doors—usually they would slide. We had not realized how strongly the pushing habit had become ingrained in us! Another new habit was sliding out of our shoes—hard on the socks. We not only learned how to ride in a jeep (it takes strong nerves and a well-padded bottom), but we passed our Korean driving test and learned to drive through the city traffic without hitting a man with a haystack on his back or a lady with a tub on her head. One day, on the way to school, we saw a woman carrying six boards on her head without using her hands. That was quite a trick, but it was topped by the lady we saw just before Christmas. She carried a five-foot evergreen in an upright flowerpot on her head, and in addition, she had a baby on her back.

We had only lived in Korea for five months before we added an orphan child to the family. She became the first of five children who lived with us at different times before going on to their new families in America. Patti was an undernourished, unloved little girl of two and a half. Our job was to get her to look and act something like a normal one-year-old child so that her new parents would not be too shocked at first sight of her. She demanded a great deal of attention and threw our entire household into confusion. When she arrived she could not walk five steps without assistance, but with encouragement and coaxing she spent more and more time on her feet. By the time she left our home she was walking, slowly and shakily, but with purpose and determination, wherever she wanted to go. At first she spent hours staring at the floor with a woebegone look that tore at our heartstrings. She would have nothing to do with any of us at close range, but she began to sob if we walked away from her. She would not go to sleep unless she was held in someone's arms or carried on the housekeeper's back. We had to teach her to sleep alone in her own bed, because we knew that her new parents would expect it. They would not know that Korean children are seldom left alone and spend most of their first two years riding on someone else's back.

Our household help was the big problem. They could not bear to hear the child cry and whenever she opened her mouth one of them was on the spot to offer her anything to stop the tears. Although we knew that they considered us mean and cruel, we enforced the rules and soon the baby learned to sleep alone and to walk alone. Within a month she had changed from a frightened and withdrawn child to one who enjoyed other people and looked for approval after each new trick. We had read of the marvelous changes that love can work in a child, but to experience it for ourselves was pure joy. We felt as if we had really accomplished something worthwhile when Patti left us for her permanent home in the United States.

Having a baby in the house again was fun for all of us too. One sunny Saturday morning I took her outside the gate to entertain her. The street was already busy, so we sat down, Korean-style, with me squatting on my haunches and Patti on my back. The Korean children in their neat gray and white uniforms and hats passed us on their way to school. Mothers with their own little ones on their backs found the American woman with a Korean baby an unusual "sight-see" and pointed at us as they discussed it. Patti amused me by pointing right back.

Two carts creaked by, piled high with shiny new church benches. One man pulled the cart and another pushed while they chanted together to coordinate their movements. Alongside ran a youth of about sixteen years. He was dressed in rags, but he wore a plastic bib around his neck and his saliva drooled out on it. Six or eight little boys kept him company, calling out to him, laughing at him, tormenting him, and just watching him. This is the fate of the "crazy ones" in Korea.

A fish merchant saw me from afar and headed for the place where we sat, hoping to make a sale. "Buy fish!" he called out, but I had no money. He carried a bowl containing about twenty different kinds of colored fish in one hand and with the other he held a basket of fish bowls in assorted sizes. I asked the price of the fish, but only so that he would stay long enough and Patti could have a closer look at the bright fish swimming in the bowl.

A child who approached us was very interested in my "pretty baby" so Patti and I walked down the street a little way with her. We stopped at the corner where a young boy was selling flowers and carrying on a heated argument with a well-dressed gentleman. When he saw us he turned to me and asked several times, "Is it not so?" But we just smiled and passed on. Three little beggar girls jumped off a step and surrounded us, tugging at my skirt and grinning out of happy, dirty faces. "Money?" they asked, in English.

"Money?" I repeated the word in Korean. "I have no money

now." A search for pockets in the skirt convinced them and they agreed that I had no money but I had a pretty baby. My dress was pretty too, they told me. They were friendly little girls.

Before we left Seoul we saw our first Korean wedding. It took place on a bitterly cold day in January in a wedding hall which was over some shops on a side street. The big room was heated with only one tiny coal stove and the people were standing three deep around it when we arrived. All the windows were open, perhaps because the stove smoked. Although I had brought my camera, my hands became too numbed to use it before the ceremony began. The bride waited in a small room in back while the rest of us shivered in the cold hall, until finally the master of ceremonies unrolled a red and white runner in the aisle and placed another runner of red silk on top of it. The guests were given paper boutonnieres and paper streamers and then the organist played the breathy processional. The bride began an unbelievably slow progress up the red carpet. She was dressed in a Western-style gown and veil, and her face was chalky white and thickly painted. Her head hung low; she was firmly supported on each side by her attendants and she looked as if she were having a very difficult time dragging her unwilling feet to the altar.

It was not a long ceremony—mercifully. He put the ring on her finger, she handed him a fountain pen, they bowed solemnly at each other once or twice, and then raced together back down the aisle while the guests pelted them with the paper ribbons and anything else within reach. We were eager to get away to a warmer place, but the couple insisted that we pose with them for an official photograph. Although it was only the second time that we had met the bride and we did not know the bridegroom at all, we obliged. But we skipped the reception.

"Time is like an allow," often says our Mr. Kim. He has learned the difference between the English "L" and "R" but he never could pronounce them right. We discovered, though, that he knows what he is talking about. Time in Korea passes so quickly that we were soon looking forward to our return to Taejon. The year in Seoul had given us only a slight familiarity with Korean language but a wide overall view of life in Korea. We had made friends with all kinds of people and we had learned from each of them. We knew what we could buy on the Korean market and we felt at ease in the Korean environment. So our second arrival at Taejon was much easier and happier than the first.

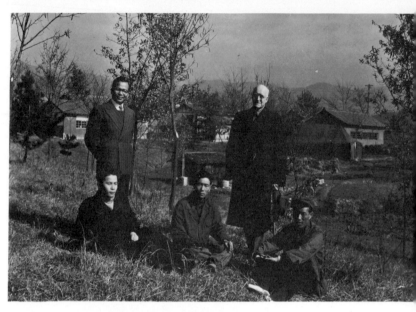

Dr. R. A. Torrey, Jr., Director of the amputee
rehabilitation program 1952-1958, with a group of
amputees on the grounds of Taejon center.

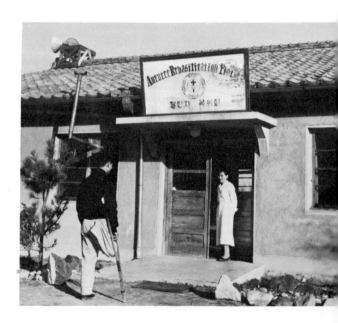

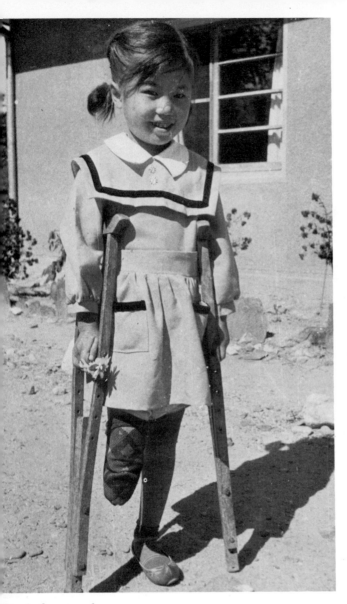

Ready for a new leg.

(opposite) A new patient arrives at the Taejon center.

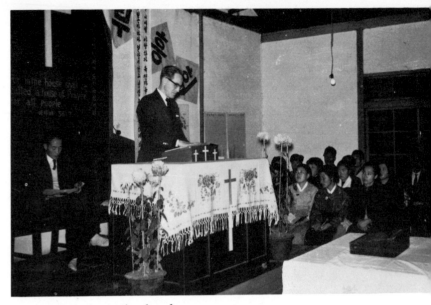

A worship service in the chapel.

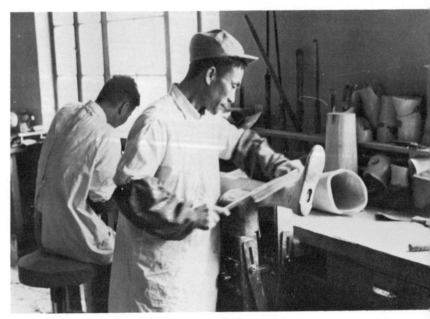

A leg amputee works on a new leg for a patient.

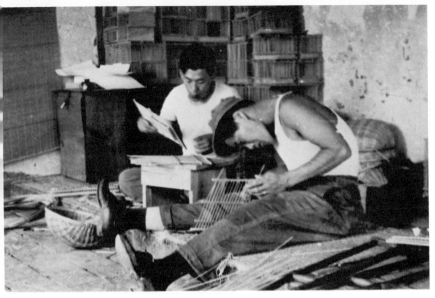

Making baskets and cages was one of the skills taught amputees.

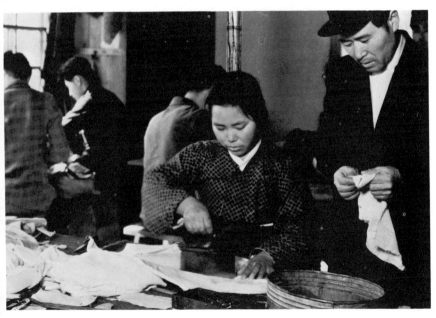

Leg amputees at work in the tailor shop.

Seoul

5

During the year we had been away, the school for missionary children at Taejon had grown. It was staffed by three teachers who had been sent out by the Southern Presbyterian Mission to spend full time, teaching the children of the missionaries. It had moved into a new building. The teaching staff was supplemented by mothers of the children—former schoolteachers—and so I too was drafted. During the years we lived in Taejon I taught typing and English and physical education to high school students. Classes were small, equipment was meager, and sometimes the school was so cold that we moved the classes home into the living room. But we learned to use every resource we could lay our hands on. We relied heavily on each other and on our imaginations and somehow, the children learned.

Dr. Torrey left Korea in the fall of 1959 and John officially assumed the position of Director at the Korea Amputee Rehabilitation Center. It was not an easy assignment to fill the shoes of a venerated missionary, especially one as beloved as Dr. Torrey. During our summer holiday, which was spent at the missionary resort on the shores of the Yellow Sea, John had let his beard grow. It was not meant to be a permanent adornment, but the Korean people at the Center were so enthusiastic about it that he postponed its removal. Since the Oriental does not usually have much facial hair, a good beard is greatly admired. It gives a man prestige and dignity, and John sorely needed all he could get of both. Our missionary friends, accustomed to individuality in its varied manifestations, admitted that John's beard gave him a vaticinal look, but the Koreans were more specific. They thought he looked exactly like the pictures of Christ. I think that John would have gotten rid of it in a hurry if it had not been possible for him to get a shave, a haircut, and a massage in the Korean barber shop for the equivalent of thirty cents in American money. A man with his own barber (and a lady barber at that!) can afford to wear a beard. The beard became a permanent part of him when he noticed that he was no longer being pointed out to others as "that man with the hooks." He had become "the man with the beard," and he appreciated the change.

While we were living in Seoul, we had become somewhat acquainted with the situation at the amputee center and had already decided that it needed some tightening up. During his last year in Korea, Dr. Torrey had become increasingly busy with arrangements for his departure. He had also declined alarmingly in health and some of the personnel at the Center had taken advantage of this situation. We were handicapped by the fact that we knew nothing of the backgrounds of the amputees who were living at the Center. So we set about getting acquainted as quickly as possible.

Many of these amputees had come to the Center because they had nowhere else to go. Some were victims of the Korean War or of hidden land mines which were left over from it. Many were children, orphaned by disease or war, or abandoned because of their disability. New cases kept coming in. One day it was a little woman who looked much older than her thirty years. She came hobbling over the hills on the uneven terrain, using only a stick and one leg. Several years before, all her toes had been amputated and a subsequent infection had resulted in a higher amputation of one leg. Because she had borne him no children, her husband had deserted her and she had long ago spent all of her money on hospitals and medicines. Could we help her? It was plain to us that this woman needed more than physical assistance.

I also remember the girl, Mi Ja, and the story she told us. She described how she had crouched motionless in a corner of a room in her brother's house, listening as her male relatives argued together about her future. For two years, since the dark day when both of Mi Ja's frostbitten feet had been amputated, her life had been completely dependent upon these men—her brothers and her uncles. Each one grudgingly gave a little money or rice for her, and her bedroll was shifted from house to house as they tired of the burden. She realized that she was even unwelcome in the home of her brother, whose children already numbered more than he could feed. Although she was always cheerful about watching the fire or mending the clothing, she bowed her head in shame before the hostile eyes of her sister-in-law when she reached for the portion of rice that was allotted to her.

Her uncle rose to speak, and when she heard his words the girl froze in horror. "It is foolish," he exclaimed, "to allow this thing to continue. A crippled woman can never hope to marry, and what good is a woman who can neither bear sons nor do any useful work? Must we forever steal food from the mouths of our children to keep this half-person alive?"

Other voices joined him. It was true that such a life was a waste, but surely they were not murderers! Mi Ja's eyes squeezed tightly shut against the angry faces, but the hot tears spilled over and fell upon her clasped hands as she waited. The men had quite forgotten her presence, as if she were already dead. Then she heard the voice of her elder brother, whom she had adored since she was old enough to recognize him.

"Mi Ja is my beloved sister," he said. "Have you ever thought about what is in her heart? I remember when she ran about through the courtyard and played jump rope with her companions. She could swing higher than all her schoolmates, and her graceful jumps on the seesaw were beautiful to watch. Now she must be carried about on another's back, like a baby, and all who see her laugh and torment her. If her life is allowed to continue in such a fashion, it would be a great unkindness to her. And what of the future? Even if it were possible for us to bear this burden for all of our lives, she is still young. And one by one we shall die. Who will feed her then?"

"Who, indeed?" inquired the others. But the elder brother held up his hand for silence.

"Mi Ja is wise," he continued. "She would neither wish to live such an unpleasant and unfruitful life, nor would she choose to make herself a weight upon the backs of others. Let us ask her mind. Surely she longs to die, and without a doubt she has already chosen for herself what method will end her sad existence."

Mi Ja held her breath and tried to make herself invisible. The men were very pleased with elder brother's speech, and they agreed to meet again in the morning to help the crippled girl to end her misery. When they had all gone out of the room, the old grandmother who helped Mi Ja to spread her bed in the corner entered it. The girl could hardly contain herself, and she confided all to the old woman.

"I do not wish to die," she had cried out brokenly against her grandmother's shoulder. "I love life, even though I have no feet. I can still hear the song of the birds when I wake in the morning, and I can see the loveliness of the azalea blooms in the courtyard. Is there no hope for me? Is one who can no longer walk good for nothing?"

The grandmother was very old and enjoyed the respect of many people. Because she was ancient and wise, everything came to her ears. She remembered the chatter of the women as they washed their clothes at the river. Someone had heard a story of a young Korean man who had lost both his hands. He had sought help from Christian missionaries, and although he was poor and could pay nothing, he had been given new hands. He had even learned a trade, so that he could return to his village as a respectable man.

And so it happened that an old woman, staggering under the weight of the husky girl on her back, had entered the Church World Service Amputee Rehabilitation Center at Taejon. They had stared around them in amazement when they came. The first sight was a group of men with iron hooks instead of hands, sitting in a shop near the entrance, making beautiful carvings. The nurse welcomed Mi Ja and her grandmother into the office. She showed Mi Ja her own artificial leg.

When John examined the stumps of her legs, Mi Ja stared at him intently. Perhaps it was the first time she had ever seen a Westerner. Certainly she had never been so close to one. He pushed gently against the flabby flesh of her stumps with his steel hooks and he felt the girl cringe away from him.

"Don't worry," he said to her, and she looked back at him uncomprehendingly, bewildered by his strange, foreign accent. "You will soon be walking again," and he smiled.

But Mi Ja did not smile. A great fear lay like a lump in her heart. She had no money at all and she knew that her family would give her no more help. She was afraid that the director would ask her to pay for her new legs.

John did not attempt an explanation. He left that up to the Korean staff who would know how to approach this girl and reassure her. It was the chaplain who explained to her that many people came to the Center for help. Some were rich and others had nothing. Some were eager to learn to care for themselves and others only sought someone to care for them so that they would not have to work. Did Mi Ja have any money at all? Could she pay a part of the cost of the new legs, or could she buy her own food while she lived at the Center and was trained to use her artificial legs?

Mi Ja threw herself at the minister's feet. "I have no money, no money at all! But I do not wish to die!" she sobbed. "I would work hard gladly if only you will allow me to stay." And then she had poured out to us her story of rejection and hopelessness.

She was trained to use a sewing machine with a hand operated wheel and she became very clever at making Western-style ladies' dresses. More and more of the Korean women were changing from the traditional *ch'ima* and *chogori* into Western styles and we hoped that Mi Ja would be able to support herself with this special skill. When she left the Center, she was given the sewing machine in order to start her own business.

Another case which came into the Center soon after our arrival was a young father—neatly dressed, clean-shaven, and freshly combed. Although he used crutches, he gave the appearance of dignity. As a prosperous merchant in Seoul, he had married the daughter of a well-to-do family and become the father of three children. But he lost his leg in an automobile accident and when he returned from the hospital he found that his house was empty. He hurried to the home of his father-in-law and inquired concerning his family. He was told that his wife wanted nothing to do with him. She felt that to be married to a cripple was beneath her, and she asked him not to return. His children, however, clung to him —one leg or two, he was their father. When he came to the Center he asked for vocational training. He had made up his mind to divorce his wife—but as we talked about it, it became apparent that the hurt in his soul was deep. Such a man needed to be given a new leg and vocational training, but he also needed to find the "balm of Gilead." It would not be good enough just to send him off with a new arm or a new leg. We began to see that we had to give these amputees more than that. We began to see the reason why we had come to Korea.

For some of the amputees there seemed to be little hope of rehabilitation. When twelve-year-old Lee Yoon Jae went with his friends to play on the mountainside, he was too young to appreciate the danger of the hand grenade that they found lying there in the long grasses. Perhaps Yoon Jae's friends were more fortunate than he . . . when the new toy exploded in their hands they died without knowing what had happened to them. Lee Yoon Jae spent long months in a mission hospital, recovering from serious burns all over his face and body. Both hands were amputated, both ears were blown off and his nose, lips, and eyelids were grotesquely scarred. His parents found him in the hospital, but they were appalled by the sight of him. They soon stopped visiting him altogether and when he was discharged he found there was no one living in the place which he had called home. No one knew what had become of his family, so at thirteen the crippled and scarred youngster was left to worry about his own future.

He was so ugly that it was hard to look at him. Even more serious, his eyelids had been burned so badly that it was impossible for him to blink and he suffered from infection in his eyes. The saliva dribbled from his misshapen lips and he continually daubed at his face with the dirty rag which he carried in one of his hook claws.

As a part of his rehabilitation, Lee was sent to a plastic surgeon who performed primary repairs on his face. His eyelids were corrected so that he could once again close his eyes and wash them out with tears. His lips were altered so that his mouth would close again, and his nose was built up to cover the gaping nostrils. Still, Lee Yoon Jae was not a normal-looking boy, so we decided to find some sheltered place where he could earn his living without fighting the stares of the crowds. He learned animal husbandry with the hope of becoming a farmer or a stock raiser.

Kim Whan Bin had lost his leg by crawling under a moving train. He came to the Church World Service Center to get an artificial leg and to learn a trade. Skin disorders among the amputees were not uncommon, especially at certain times of the year when the weather became cold and water and soap were scarce. So Kim's dormitory mates laughed and teased him about his complaints and told him to go and get a bath.

After Kim had been examined by three different doctors, it was no longer a laughing matter. The boy had leprosy. Arrangements were made to have him admitted to the leprosy clinic where a missionary doctor promised to look after him. We were happy that the disease had been discovered at its beginning, so that it could be arrested before permanent disfigurement took place. But Kim Whan Bin did not see it that way. His mind was still clouded with the old superstitious fears of leprosy and its implications of banishment, mutilation, and decay. He refused to believe that he had leprosy. Like an ostrich that hides its head in the sand, he simply shut out the possibility that he could have this disease and he refused to be treated for it. To each suggestion that we made he would shake his head and reply stubbornly, "It is not true. It is not leprosy."

And so he had to be dismissed from the Center. He went back to his home, or perhaps he continued to wander. We never found out whether he told his family what had happened or whether he waited until the signs of leprosy became so unmistakable that they were visible to others and he could no longer ignore them. We do not know what happened to Kim Whan Bin; we never saw him again.

Not all of the patients came to the amputee center. One day we were asked by a pastor to visit the home of a lad who had lost his leg just a few weeks previously. We found the home about one hundred yards from the end of the road where we had to leave the car. As we threaded our way up the muddy path through front yards, backyards, and alleys, we were followed by a rapidly-growing crowd of men, women, children, and dogs. The house we sought was occupied by four families, with the crippled youth's family of six persons living together in one room. People were everywhere. The visit of a foreign woman and a foreign man with iron hands caused more excitement in that neighborhood than the boy had created by losing his leg. The amputee crawled out onto the porch and John examined his stump. While this was going on, the amputee center pastor took advantage of the opportunity to bring a brief evangelistic message to the people who pressed closely around us. Both the boy and his family were greatly encouraged when they heard that we expected the amputee to be walking again in a few months' time.

Through the love and generosity of Christians in American churches, we were able to enroll this same boy in school. Later on, when we paid a courtesy call at the home to compliment the mother upon her son's progress we found her pale and sick. She confided that she had visited a doctor but he had recommended surgery which she could not possibly afford. Her face lit up as she explained to us that everything would be all right. "Jesus gives me strength," she said.

She had been attending church since our first visit, and she thanked God for the blessings which had come to her since our first meeting with her. We asked her if she would accept our offer to go to the Jesus Hospital, which is run by the Southern Presbyterian Mission at Chunju, about sixty-five miles from Taejon. A week later, after the surgery, she was very low. With her son, who attended the services in our chapel, we prayed that the Lord would spare this woman's life in order that she might be a witness to her unbelieving neighbors who had advised her against turning her back on the ancient Chinese doctors and their remedies. Although she had cancer, she was able to return home to her family and she used the remainder of her life witnessing, telling her neighbors of the joy that she had found in knowing Christ.

In another home, we found a family of five living in one tiny room. In one corner lay our patient, a young man of twenty-one years. He had attended college for three years, but after the death of his father, the situation of the family had declined. At one time the boy had been a church member, but he had lost his faith while attending college, as so many do. After losing both legs in an accident, he had become utterly despondent and discouraged. On both his legs we found several large, draining sores and the young man told us that twice each week a doctor's apprentice came in to give him "shots" and to change the dressings on the legs. The boy seemed to have no interest in recovery, since the future held no hope for him as an amputee.

We spoke to him and his family about Christ's love for them. We told him that the love of God in the hearts of his children made them concerned about one another. The boy listened respectfully, and later he wrote us a letter in English which was kept in our files at the Center. He said:

> By good graces of the respectable director and the staff at the Center, I have safely arrived in Chunju, Jesus Hospital, and am receiving medical treatment. How are you since I saw you last? I feel that I am in a dream now as I am looking back about myself because I had no idea to be rehabilitated my disability. But now, fortunately, God has called me and led me to you for rehabilitating my disabled body. I will not forget your kindness of helping me forever. Of course, I will tell you about my gratitude in detail when I return back to there, but I write this brief and hasty writing to expressing my gratitude toward your help.
>
> During these days I am researching the Christian catechism and praying God in my mind. Now I believe that I am cleansed from my sin by the blood of Jesus Christ because I believe in God. Please do not forget to lead me into the deep Christian life.

The mother and sister of this boy are still in regular attendance at the local Presbyterian church. The last we heard of him, the boy himself intended to finish college and prepare for the ministry.

Experiences such as these soon taught us that the work of

rehabilitation involved much more than the careful building and fitting of artificial limbs or the training in the use of them. It involved much more than the teaching of a vocation to handicapped people. The Taejon amputee center had been the answer to an emergency situation, but the amputees kept coming. In addition to the old war cases, people came with amputations from accidents, from disease or neglect, from snakebite, or through ignorance and quack medicine. It became obvious that few of these disabled were able to make an adjustment to their handicap and that giving them a new arm or a new leg was not the whole answer to their problems. They faced a hostile society and a lifetime of rejection.

Thus, recognition of the need of wider rehabilitation service gradually developed. It seemed to us that these disabled people needed professional assistance which must involve several different services. A hungry person can be given food . . . but this does not help him for long. Tomorrow he will be hungry again. An artificial limb may help a man to walk, but it cannot solve his emotional needs or restore him to his family. Our service to the disabled must include the whole man—his emotional and spiritual needs as well as his physical need.

We began to experiment with new ideas. It was uphill work. During the seven years the Center had existed the staff and the amputees had developed habit patterns which were difficult to break. We did not know exactly how to proceed, and we made mistakes. But we found the challenge exciting and we began to see the goal ahead. The most difficult part of the task would be to make others see it too and understand the direction in which we wanted to move. And so we began our program of public education.

6

The new era at the Taejon amputee center began with the erection of new office quarters on the Center grounds. During the years of his administration, Dr. Torrey had used an office which adjoined his residence in the city of Taejon, about three miles from the Center itself. We found that it was impossible to run the Center effectively from such a distance. In the new building was a dispensary, where weekly clinics gave us direct contact with the trainees. There was also the office of the social worker, where the personal problems of the clients were handled. Slowly, confidence in the office staff developed, but not without problems and casualties. We sought to exchange comfortable habits for habits which we considered more effective, to do the right thing without regard for personal interests or ambitions, and to work for the common good rather than for that of a favored few.

Many of the staff members in the vocational training shops had maintained the ancient method of teaching—by apprenticeship. We spent months in the reorganization of each department, trying to set them up for classroom-type instruction with a progressive pattern of training. We tried to check the progress of each trainee and to set a definite date for the completion of the course. A check among the trainees disclosed that some of them had been in one department for periods of one to five years without completing any specific part of the training. These trainees were grouped into classes according to skill, and monthly reports on their progress were kept in the office. Several trainees were discharged because they had shown no aptitude for any of the vocational programs which we had to offer. This was traumatic, both for the amputee and for the director. The person who faced discharge sometimes became hysterical and wept and beat his head against the wall. He would tell us that if we put him out of the shelter of the amputee center we would be throwing him to the wolves. He could do nothing but starve outside. Such experience convinced the director that the goal of rehabilitating the handicapped people who had come to the Center had not been achieved. They had been fed and clothed and sheltered from the pressures which others face in the world, but they had never learned to accept themselves as they were and to live with their handicaps.

There were several changes which we wanted to make immediately. All of the buildings, which had been intended as temporary structures, needed immediate repairs. Some had reached the stage where it was hardly worthwhile to invest money in repairing them. They had been constructed with pressed-earth blocks, into which the rats had tunneled to make their homes, weakening the walls. Many of the foundations and walls had cracked, and floors were rotted and dangerous for people who walked with crutches or artificial legs. The chapel building was used every day of the week as a training room and in the evenings for recreation. It was impossible to heat, and birds flew in and out during the church service and settled above our heads on the rafters. In the summertime, swarms of kamikaze June bugs swooped toward the naked light bulbs which hung down from their cords, and this distracted both audience and speaker. Our Korean friends decided that a ceiling in the chapel would be a great improvement, but they disagreed with us about screens on the windows, insisting that screens would make the building too hot inside. They shut out the air. So the windows remained open in the summertime. We often had to open them in the winter also because of smoke and fumes from the three little coal-burning stoves which were kept stoked in an optimistic attempt to heat the barn-like auditorium.

Careful planning and disciplined spending, increased efficiency and a slightly reduced patient load—with more careful study of the patients we already had—reduced the operational costs considerably. We soon learned that some of our amputees had parents and homes of their own, and we could see no reason to continue boarding such students. A number of the amputees who had been living at the Center for a long time indicated that they had no real desire for rehabilitation. They refused to work and spent their time loafing on the streets of the city or inside the dormitories at the Center. It was quite a shock to these people when they were asked to leave. They had assumed that Christianity was a religion of love, and no one had ever explained to them that love always includes discipline.

It became clear that although we could teach a person to weave baskets out of bamboo or to make pails out of tin, we must also teach him how to run his business if we expected him to make a living at it. The sheltered workshops were not the place to do this. So some of the amputees were given "on-the-job" training; they were apprenticed to shops outside with the amputee center assuming the responsibility for their wages over a period of time. After that time, the owner of the shop was given the opportunity to hire the trainee. We had nothing to lose by such an arrangement. The wages of the trainee cost us no more than his room and board would have cost if he stayed at the Center. He was trained to please the owner of the establishment and if the trainee was unsuccessful, the owner himself lost face. In this way, many of the amputees were placed on jobs outside in the workaday world and scratched from our permanent rolls.

Sometimes the amputee himself was not as great a problem as his family. I remember the mother who came in with her son. While the boy stood silently by, his mother wept loudly and told her story of woe.

"He is such a good boy! His teachers always praised him; his friends all loved him; the neighbors spoke well of him and blessed his future. I was so proud of my son. I cannot believe that this has happened to him."

The boy hung his head, empty sleeves dangling at his sides. It was hard to imagine him as a friendly, lovable person. But it was not hard to understand his hostility as his mother continued to talk.

"The gods hate us," she said. "Somehow we have sinned, and

this is our punishment." The mother, a widow in her mid-fifties, was a farmer. Since the death of her husband several years before, she had been the main breadwinner of the family, and her pride and her future were in her three growing sons. This boy, a good-looking lad of seventeen years, had fallen off a moving train on his way to school six months before.

Our job would be to teach this young man to accept his handicap before we could teach him to overcome it. He must want to take his place among normal people, to compete with them on their terms. He had cut himself off from neighbors and friends in his bitterness against his fate and he was now all alone in his misery.

As soon as his artificial limbs were ready, he tried them on. They were heavy and clumsy on his unaccustomed stumps, and he was ready to discard them immediately. But a period of training was required before he could be discharged and so, living with other amputees, watching them as they performed skilled tasks that most people with two hands and two feet had not learned to do, the new arrival gradually forgot that he was disabled. His bitterness was met with patience, for a man who had lost his own leg or arm could understand the hurt that lies in the heart of another. The boy learned to know God too, and God's love for man. Here, in this place, he saw Christian people who showed their love for God by the love and service that they gave to others. The fact that the Director, who was himself a double arm amputee, took pride in his mastery of the artificial arms and hooks that he wore, impressed the boy. He began to practice with his hooks and was eager to demonstrate each new accomplishment. He made friends who encouraged and spurred him on with their examples and their challenges.

After the boy had lived at the rehabilitation center for two months, his mother came to visit him. He was thrilled by the prospect of demonstrating his independence to her. His face shone as he entered the office where she waited. His step was jaunty and the new arms swung carelessly as he walked. She could not know that each casual swing was deliberate and practiced!

Crying out that she had missed him, the mother ran toward him. But the son, eager to show his new arms, hardly heard her.

He was full of news about his new life. He told her about the pig that he was raising to take home with him, and about the plans to raise more livestock on the farm. He told her about his new friends, forgetting to mention the fact that each of them was missing one or two limbs. His mother listened in amazement, and stared at the artificial arms the boy was wearing. Grinning mischievously, he pinched her ear with his hook and laughed aloud as she smiled back at him.

Some parents gave us more trouble. We had been treating a little five-year-old girl who had been bitten by a snake while her parents worshiped at a Buddhist shrine on the hillside. The family was very poor and so we hired them to work in the kitchen and dining hall at the Center. We believe that, if it is at all possible, people who receive help should make some effort to pay for it, even if it is only a token payment. This enables them to hang on to a vestige of self-respect, and self-respect is important if you have been forced to live on the charity of others for a long time. The child's mother was a humble, hard-working woman, but her father had a problem with drink. Sometimes he beat his wife and the two little girls.

One day he disappeared, taking both children with him. The mother was heartbroken. She realized that he had taken the crippled child and her little sister in order to force them to beg and earn a living for the three of them that way. There was nothing we could do or say to comfort the poor mother. One evening some of the staff and student amputees were sitting together with her in her room, talking of her misfortune. As they had done before, they prayed with her for the return of her children. While they prayed, the dog began to bark outside. Shortly after, the two little ones appeared at the door, hand in hand. The father had decided that the care of two children was not worth what they could bring in by begging, so he had abandoned them and they had found their own way back to their mother's home.

In some cases, the poverty of the amputee's family made acceptance and rehabilitation almost impossible. If the amputee himself was the breadwinner, he had probably come to us after a period of hospitalization which had already exhausted the economic resources of the entire clan. Of course we could not, in cases such as that, limit our help to the patient alone. We had to extend our concern to the rest of the family too, since this, and not his own recovery, would be our patient's primary concern. Recognition for wider rehabilitation service developed gradually. When a man came to our Center asking for a new leg, we had to recognize the fact that he might be the sole support of his family. We knew that he could not be expected to cooperate wholeheartedly in our effort to help him if he was distracted by anxiety for the welfare of his wife and children.

If a child was brought in with a missing arm, the handicap was only a small part of the problem. In many cases, the family was looking for someone to take the burden and disgrace of the disabled child off their hands. When we had taught a young amputee to walk or to feed himself again, what could we offer him in the future? If he had nothing to look forward to but discrimination and prejudice, what had we gained by fitting him with an artificial limb? The need for qualified social workers thus became obvious to us very soon and we began to make plans to change the Taejon Vocational Rehabilitation Center to point it toward the goal of total rehabilitation.

In the beginning, we sought to improve the quality of the products which were being turned out by the various vocational training shops, with the hope of selling these products outside and earning some income. In this way we thought we could not only improve the skills of the amputees but also teach them profit and loss. We contacted outlets in Seoul and offered our samples to the ladies' auxiliary of the United States Army and Aid organization. The goods were displayed at their annual bazaar and one hundred dollars' worth was sold within a few hours. We could have sold much more if we had been more optimistic in our preparations. The amputees were elated by this success, but in figuring up their accounts they learned something about business procedure. They had counted the cost of materials, but they had completely overlooked such items as overhead and wages. This is the danger in a sheltered workshop situation. The purpose of rehabilitation is not profit-seeking: rehabilitation, in terms of dollars and cents, never expects to break even. But in order to prepare our trainees for independence and to live outside the subsidy of the Center, we had to teach them the facts of life also.

Our own training had been in an environment where consultation was readily available. Advice and expert help were at hand for any sort of exigency. We had come to a place where we, as strangers, had to assume complete responsibility for the life and conduct of people who had been forced by circumstances into habits of lawlessness, indolence, begging, and dependence. They had become undisciplined, and years of suppression, poverty, and war had taught them deception and distrust. Many amputees had come to the Center seeking only shelter, with no motivation at all toward rehabilitation. Korean society, in general, offered them neither sympathy nor understanding. Having suffered in the past from the desperation of cripples who banded together to force an indifferent public to notice them and give them food or money, people responded to the sight of an amputee with fear or hostility.

Could we, as foreigners, appreciate the mental anguish and the physical suffering which had been the lot of these people? The process of rebuilding their lives required much more skill and training than we possessed. The facilities for carrying out this work needed an atmosphere which would permit freedom and yet allow for the administration of rules. We had to eliminate the irresponsible habits and at the same time develop the confidence of our patients.

Social service cannot exist in isolation. It is dependent upon a wider group and it must be part of the group. Consultation and advice must be readily available from other members of the group. Opportunities for specialized training and job placement must be available to encourage the skeptical amputee. And so, by the time we had been working at the amputee center in Taejon for a year, we had already decided that the project should be moved to Seoul. There was a great deal of criticism on this decision, which was not unexpected. In Korea, all roads lead to Seoul, and many fought this tendency to make the whole country into a one-city nation. But we felt that in the work of rehabilitation, as we visualized it, there was little choice. Rehabilitation is a phase of medicine which is still not wholly accepted, even in the United States of America. A constant program of public education is necessary to remind employers and the general public of the important role the handicapped are able to play in society. Doctors, therapists, counselors, social workers must work together in joint effort to promote the cause. We believed that the amputee project could lead the way in Korea for those who had other handicaps to develop an effective program of rehabilitation.

7

The decision to move the amputee center to Seoul had been based on sober reflection. We had no desire to leave Taejon, which we had found a most pleasant place to live. Looking back upon our comfortable home there and the good friends and neighbors we enjoyed, we still feel nostalgia. We will always be grateful to the Southern Presbyterian and the Southern Baptist Missions for renting houses on their compounds to us and sharing their fellowship with us. Not only did this enable us to live closer to the amputee center, but it also gave us the benefit of living close to the mission school which the children attended. They could play with friends who lived next door and they could roam the wooded hills without fear or danger. The usual worries which American parents have about letting their teen-agers or little ones walk out alone were unknown to us in Taejon. Although we had to take precaution against impure water and parasites in food bought on the market, we benefited from the absence of smog in the open country and we did not miss the city traffic. We ate fresh vegetables from our own gardens, strawberries in season, apples from the nearby orchards, and we butchered pigs which had been fattened on our own garbage.

Some missionaries complain about the enforced closeness of the compound community, but we looked upon it as a blessing. The concern of our neighbors was not nosyness, but a genuine Christian love. They were willing to help us in large or small emergencies;

we shared our joys and sorrows and friends and children; we worked together and we worshiped together. To a family of Yankees in a settlement of Southerners, it was a warm experience. For our children, who had been born into the tightly-knit, provincial Dutch settlements of Michigan, it was enriching to have friends from different backgrounds.

One of our cooperative ventures in the community was a servicemen's "retreat" which was organized by Bob Floyd, a Southern Presbyterian Army chaplain who often visited in our home at Taejon. He had found the peace of country living and the fellowship of kindred souls so refreshing after the regimentation and routine of the Army camps, the barrenness of the Korean countryside around the Demilitarized Zone, and the lack of anything homelike in the life of the American soldier stationed in Korea, that he wanted to share it with his men. The mission community responded and offered to meet the men at the Taejon train station, billet them among the various homes, and entertain them for the weekend. Each home hosted two to four soldiers. On Saturday evening we held a community spaghetti supper in the school dining room and all had an opportunity to meet one another. The names of the GI guests were put into a hat and each mission family drew out two new names for Sunday night supper. In this way the men were redistributed among the various homes and were able to meet a different family and to visit another missionary home. After supper on Sunday there was a community sing and coffee.

The thirty-three men who made the first trip were so enthusiastic in their thanks that Chaplain Floyd began planning another excursion. All of the men who had come the first time signed up again, but the word had gotten around and they were "bumped" by forty-two others who wanted to try a taste of missionary life.

Another venture in which we all took part was not so pleasant. The principal of the mission school, who lived in a few rooms in the school building, had acquired a darling, dumpy puppy for his baby daughter. Playing with this dog became a favorite recreation for the kindergarten and first-grade children and even for the pre-schoolers who came to the building for Sunday school classes. When the dog died, suddenly and under suspicious circumstances, all the children grieved. But when the principal called an emergency meeting of parents to inform us that the reports from the Army laboratory had confirmed his suspicions that the dog had died with rabies, there was consternation. The Army medical unit had followed through by advising the parents of all children who had had any contact with the pup to come to the base in Taejon for a series of preventive inoculations. We were spared nothing. The Army medical officer informed us in detail that the shots were painful, that each child would have to endure one every day for fourteen consecutive days, and that any child who had an allergy to eggs could be in more trouble from the shots than from the rabies. But there was little choice, so parents grimly made plans to transport fifty-one people, including most of our children who ranged in age from two through twelve, three miles to the Army base every day as soon as the classes were finished at school.

Every day the mission Land Rovers lined up in formation, with the youngsters fighting for the best seats. At first many of them howled and cowered, but within a few days most had become casual about the trip and treated it as a nuisance that they had to get over with as quickly as possible.

The shots were given in the abdomen and my sympathy for the kids grew with each new welt. Our son Dirk's tummy looked like a flower garden after the first week. Since the U.S. Army is humane and tenderhearted too, the medics were more disturbed by what they had to do to those little ones than the children themselves were. Each day they prepared a surprise for them: the first day it was lollipops, the second day, bubble gum. For missionary children who did not share the delights of the PX, these were rare treats and they looked forward to the daily gifts. But after the first week, even this pleasure wore thin and the children as well as their parents became bored with the whole procedure. The ride to the city, the quick passing of the long line through the dispensary—it all became a tedious duty and everyone, including the medics, was relieved when at last it was over.

There was a certain amount of the excitement and challenge of frontier living in the life at Taejon. The unexpected could always happen and often did. One day our routine was turned upside down by the arrival of a TV director and his crew who made a documentary film for American audiences. Then there was the fun of receiving letters from people in various parts of the United States who had viewed the film. Another film director made a very fine movie for U.S. Information Service about the rehabilitation of an amputee at the Taejon Vocational Center. The activities and presence of this film crew enlivened the Center for weeks.

There were also the crises . . . the day I returned home from work at the Center to be met by an excited crowd of children with the news that Joy had been bitten by a dog and was all bloody. Going into the house, I could hear Joy screaming. I met Mary in tears and found Mr. Kim so nervous and scared that he could scarcely speak. He had Joy's hand bandaged up so that I couldn't tell how bad the wound was, but I saw the blood on the bandages. (Mr. Kim didn't wash it; he just covered it up.) Just as everyone began to calm down, in rushed the lady who owned the dog. She was also in tears. We had to calm her down before we could all go to the Baptist compound next door to see the nurse. When the nurse uncovered Joy's hand, I felt like a fool. The skin was hardly broken. A few Band-Aids after a good washing would have taken care of it.

The time that Mary fell into the pit of night soil was less frightening but harder to live down. We saw her coming, reeking and rueful, carrying one dripping boot in her hand. Since we were entertaining guests in the living room, I steered her to the back of the house, but it was no good. Although Mary was bathed at least three times with hot water and laundry soap, she still made a strong impression at the dinner table.

One day, while I was alone in the house, I watched a three-foot red and black snake slither over the doorsill into the bathroom. I didn't know how to handle that situation, but the snake took care of itself. Within a minute or two, it slid out again, back into the garden. We had all kinds of guests in those days.

Our greatest worry was the lack of adequate medical facilities in Taejon. As director of the amputee center, my husband was often called upon to make life-and-death decisions. Neither of us had any medical training and we felt our responsibilities keenly when we received calls from the Center asking us what to do in case of a sick trainee. The nearest dependable hospital was at Chunju, a two-hour train ride. Most of the Korean people hosted worms, and the symptoms of worms were often alarming. We had to decide whether our patients were suffering from acute indigestion, from an attack by the worms, or from a ruptured appendix.

One evening John received an emergency telephone call. The head man in the bamboo training shop had gone out of his mind. He was foaming at the mouth, babbling incoherently, and thrashing about on the floor. What could we do?

I don't know what a psychiatrist or a physican would have done in that situation, but I remembered a movie in which the zoo keeper used a tranquilizer gun to catch a wild animal which had broken out of its cage. So I offered my tranquilizers. We gave the disturbed man two tranquilizers and a sleeping pill and hoped for the best. He slept for two days and woke up refreshed and behaving normally. He did not even remember his fit.

More memorable was the afternoon I returned from a trip into the city to find a suicide on the front porch. John had gone off to America for five weeks and I had just reached the point where I did not think I could carry the double load of responsibilities another day. As I drove into the compound gate, I had only one thought in my mind—taking a hot bath and collapsing into bed. But before the car reached our driveway, it was intercepted by our cook who stood in the middle of the road, wildly waving his arms. Wearily, I stopped and leaned my head out of the window.

Mr. Kim was too excited to speak clearly. And I was too tired to get excited, even after I had grasped his message. It seemed that one of our women amputees had decided to end her life dramatically and publicly by drinking lye. This young woman had given us a great deal of trouble already. She had become infatuated with the male arm amputee who was working for us as gardener, and she announced that she had conceived a child by him. Our reaction was very Western and we thought everything would be solved if the couple could marry. But the boy was reluctant. He said very little, and did not refuse to participate in the ceremony but it was obvious that he had no desire for it. He neither admitted nor denied his paternity but seemed detached from the whole mess. One of our Korean co-workers quietly began to investigate the lady's past and offered the information that she was already married. She had run away from her mother-in-law's home, taking with her all the money she found in the house. Confronted with this information, the girl became stormy and threatened to get an abortion. Once again, we reacted as American Christians and astonished our Korean friends.

"Do you really feel that abortion is sin?" a deacon in the Korean Presbyterian Church had asked. "It is quite common in Korea. The wives of our Elders have abortions."

Mr. Steensma had been quite shocked by this information. He definitely believed that abortion was sin. "But," timidly asked a Korean Christian, "if your wife does not have abortions, how is it that you have only four children?"

As it turned out, the amputee girl did not need an abortion. She had lied about her pregnancy in an effort to snare another husband. But she had lost face and was expelled in disgrace from the Center. She had now chosen our home for her suicide demonstration because the man who had rejected her was our employee.

I did not know what to do. So I went for help to our nearest neighbor. Keith had an excellent command of Korean language and enough prestige in the Korean community so that I knew he could help me. When he came over and looked at the girl as she lay writhing and moaning on the floor of the veranda, he shook his head.

"I think she is faking," he announced. "But we can't take a chance on it. Let's put her in the Rover and take her in to the hospital." Together with the cook and the gardener, we lifted the squirming woman into the back of the Rover. Her groans were pitiful, but nobody in the crowd showed sympathy. Life is cheap in Korea and this girl belonged to no one. She was a cripple and she had decided to remove herself. That was all there was to it. She meant nothing, even as a human being to those who looked on.

In the emergency room of the dingy government hospital to which Keith drove us, attendants prepared to pump out the woman's stomach. When they began to slide the tube down her throat she suddenly changed her story and loudly protested that she had actually taken no lye at all. She was terrified and begged the hospital attendants to let her go. Keith calmly discussed her case with the Korean doctors.

"We can't take a chance," he said. "She may be lying because she is afraid of the hospital. Better to be on the safe side, now that she's here, and pump the stomach."

We left the girl on the table, and, as we walked back out to the Land Rover, Keith grinned wickedly and remarked with some satisfaction, "She won't try that again."

Whether she did or not, we never knew. We did not hear from the girl after that.

The lack of sympathy shown by the Korean people toward the unfortunates in their society shocked me. But the sentimentality and undirected sympathy with which the American community indulged themselves was an even greater burden. Several years before our arrival in Korea, a beggar child was brought to the amputee rehabilitation center. The boy was half frozen and caked with dirt, and both legs had been taken off below the knees by a train accident. He was fitted with artificial legs and trained to use them. He was cleaned and clothed and cared for, and soon he was running and jumping around and attending the regular elementary school nearby.

Supported by regular donations from interested friends abroad, it would seem that his future was well taken care of. The boy was an excellent prospect for complete rehabilitation. But he ran away.

Why did he run away? The answer is easy. After two or three years of regulated living he began to long for the freedom and companionship of his former wandering life. The beggars in Korea, like beggars everywhere, have their own society and it is a closed brotherhood. Our boy had forgotten the disadvantages of begging, and he remembered only the excitement, the sense of belonging, the adventure. He could no longer feel the cold and the pangs of hunger, but he was chafing under the discipline and duty of being a schoolboy.

He decided to go back into the clan of beggars and to be his own master once again. We searched for him, but we could not find him. At last we had to write to his sponsor and ask him if he would consider supporting a different child.

This was not a new experience for us. Beggar boys often rejoined the fraternity after a few months or years. They are the real-life Huck Finns of Korea.

Sometime later, a U.S. government employee appeared at our offices in Seoul with a little boy of about the same age. He, too, was a double leg amputee so he appeared to be an ideal replacement for the lad who had run away.

His sponsor told us a pitiful story of how she had found the child crawling over the pavements of Seoul. She had taken him to her apartment, bathed and fed him and showered him with love. She bought him new clothing in the PX to replace his vermin-filled rags and now she wanted to buy artificial legs for the poor boy.

Fortunately, she had come to the right place. Although there were many places in Seoul where she could have bought artificial appliances, most of the prostheses were badly fitted and poorly constructed, so that they did an amputee more harm than good. They often caused painful pressure sores which eventually broke down the tissues of the stump and often made reamputation necessary.

The kind lady was not seeking charity. She asked for the best that money could buy and she was willing to pay for it out of her own salary. She offered to pay all the boy's expenses, including room and board, physical and occupational therapy. She even had dreams of specialized vocational training, or perhaps of sending her boy through college.

When she brought the child in, he turned out to be none other than our own little runaway. He had sold his newly-made artificial legs and was back at the bottom rung of his old profession when the lady found him and befriended him.

Now the cycle had begun anew. The woman was even more surprised than we were when the identity of her protégé was disclosed. She had believed every word of the story the boy had given her. And why not? He looked destitute and helpless enough. We were happy that we were able to save this generous woman from disappointment, heartache, and needless expense, but her story is not unique. Many, many foreigners have been used and abused simply because of their tender hearts, their ignorance, and gullibility. Some of them prefer it this way. They enjoy playing Santa Claus . . . or is it God?

Time after time we could read in the papers about well-intentioned GIs or do-gooders who suddenly saw a need in Korea and decided to fill it. They did not know or did not want to know of the many qualified organizations which were already there to care for those needs. Well-trained personnel who are familiar with the problems of the country to which they have been sent and are experienced in dealing with them are standing ready to help. Yet they are often ignored. Hometown newspapers build a good human interest story out of the letter which pleads for used clothing or toys for children, and hometown people respond so generously that the well-meaning Santa in Korea is unable to distribute the overflow of gifts wisely. Much of it then finds its way into the black market. Some foreigners overseas like to take stray children as pets or mascots, with the best of intentions, no doubt, but with no idea of what effect such an unnatural existence has on the future of the child. Many of the pro-tem parents return to their own country and never follow through on the child, leaving him emotionally scarred and unable to drop back into his own society.

We cannot condemn people for being good and generous. But none of us should take our role as the steward of God's gifts too lightly. Our duty is to give, but also to take the time and make the effort to investigate needs. It is all too easy to succumb to emotion and to close our eyes to facts. It is good that Christian hearts are moved by stories and pictures of emaciated people who plead for mercy with their sunken, suffering eyes. It is good that Christian love responds to the plight of children who must live under bridges or in caves. But a little thinking is enough to tell us that relief is only the beginning of the story. If we truly care for the unfortunate one as a person, we must investigate the background of his need. We must lend our support to those agencies which we know are reliable and which are working toward the purpose which we, as individuals, would like to accomplish.

Perhaps missionaries themselves are to blame for the distorted picture that the people in America have of the work of mercy which goes on among underprivileged peoples. We have presented our cause in the mistaken belief that a calculated appeal to the emotions is the *only* way to get a donation. We have forgotten that to a Christian, sharing is a natural response to the outpouring of God's blessing in our lives. To a Christian, a brother's need is an opportunity. We do not want to give from a sense of shame or from a sense of duty. We want to express our gratitude by our giving. We want to show our love, as God has shown his love for us.

If we would tell you about the lives which have already been restored, if we would show you that those whom you have already helped by your gifts are now giving their own lives to the service of their fellowmen, if we present to you healthy children and happy parents, would you prefer such an approach to the pathetic pictures of neglected human beings which have stirred you in the past? It is true that the church must feed the hungry, clothe the naked, heal the sick, restore usefulness to the blind and the lame; but the church is not fulfilling this ministry when it does superficial work. The church must also be prepared to deal with the complexity and variety of problems that confront the work of Christian mercy in foreign societies or in unchurched countries.

Christ's example is plain enough. The church has the potential to make an impact upon needy people. But such a mission is surely worthy of our best talent and of more coordinated planning between the clergy and the laity, between denominations and their Boards, and the representatives of the Boards overseas. We must not leave this work to amateurs.

8

At the close of his first two years as director of amputee rehabilitation for Korea Church World Service, John Steensma submitted his ideas for reorganization of the Center and his reasons for it in a special report to the National Council of Churches in the U.S.A., to the World Council of Churches in Geneva, and to concerned missionary representatives in Korea. This report not only reflected the conclusions which he had reached after two years of working in the rehabilitation center at Taejon, Korea, but it showed the result of fifteen previous years of conditioning by leaders and authorities in the field of rehabilitation.

He had called upon his past experience in his new post, and he had found that some of the rules which applied in America caused conflict in Korea. He had evaluated and tested various approaches while he sought to carry on established practices. He had sounded out new ideas, then discarded them for others. The responsibility to thousands of people who contributed to this work of mercy through their church offerings and who expected him to administer their funds toward the best interests of the Korean amputees weighed heavily on him. He realized that the attitudes and habits of Korean amputees in the future would depend upon the success or failure of teaching them to live with their handicaps. This adjustment to society—not prosthetic fitting and vocational training by themselves—became the important responsibility of the rehabilitation center whenever an amputee was admitted.

John was very much aware that the story of the Taejon center community, with its tragic simplicity, had great appeal as a fundraising gimmick. He had already learned that people respond with compassion to the sight of a person who was filthy, crippled, hopeless, and helpless. They were touched to see that same person raised up on two legs, clean-shaven, and dressed in clean clothing, walking about with a smile on his face. This was a daily story at the amputee project. The amputee was well cared for and happy with other people who had similar disabilities. His adjustment to people who shared his problem was simple. Co-trainees were sympathetic, and instructors were understanding—to a fault. There was no discrimination, no need to compete at the Taejon Amputee Rehabilitation Center.

This Center represented the initial phase of rehabilitation. But rehabilitation cannot stop there. Such a framework gradually undermines the purpose of sound rehabilitation practice. It teaches a cripple dependence upon a sheltered community and increases the difficulty of returning to a normal environment. The same principle holds true for leprosy colonies, widows' homes, orphanages, and similar institutions which isolate people from society.

A survey of more than eighty amputees who had been "rehabilitated" at the Taejon center from its beginning until it was closed in 1962 provided an eye opener for our Korean social worker and converted him to the concept of "total rehabilitation." The clients in the survey had received medical services, prosthetic fitting, training in the use of their new limbs, vocational training. The majority had also received baptism and admission to the church.

These former patients were all sought out and located in their homes and villages. The results were surprising and upsetting, but they bore out our conviction that, although the Taejon center had served many in a physical way and had changed the lives of some, there was need for a new approach. Of the more than eighty persons visited, only five were productive. Interestingly, these five were also active Christians, serving their community and church. The other seventy-five ex-patients had reverted to their old patterns of dependency. Few of them were wearing their prostheses and they had withdrawn from the society in which they lived. The majority had returned to the traditional religious ideas and practices which were a part of their family lives. All expressed the hope of being readmitted to the new Center at Seoul as soon as it could be built!

This experience was enough to convince Kim Young Hyuk, who served as assistant director and social work supervisor for the Center, that what had been called rehabilitation was not rehabilitation at all. He realized that a piecemeal restoration of the individual would not do, but that a complexity of services would be needed to treat the whole man. This process must begin, if possible, at the time of the injury and loss and continue through the time when the client would secure gainful employment.

Many reasons might be given to account for the results of that particular survey. The economic conditions in Korea during those years and the complete instability of the political and governmental structure are partly responsible. The culture and structure of society impeded acceptance of "abnormal" members. To some extent, the "survival of the fittest" psychology still exists in Korea, especially in the remote areas of the country.

But these reasons did not alter the fact that the Center in Taejon had provided little stimulus to the handicapped or to the rest of the Korean people to change the existing situation. It simply offered the amputee both short-term and long-term relief from rejection. It made no effort to determine the causes of rejection, since there was no contact with the family members of the disabled person. It was almost impossible to obtain a true picture of social background or personal history of any case. Except for the usual citations and awards for humanitarian services which were conferred regularly upon foreign directors of relief projects, the Korean government took little notice of our work. It was obvious to everyone that the government could not possibly take over the management and support of the many welfare projects which had been initiated and promoted by foreign agencies. Therefore, it was up to us either to assure the support of these institutions forever or to take steps to dissolve them and get the inmates back into society.

A third, but more difficult choice would be to convince organizations of individuals in Korean society to assume the responsibility for the continuance of rehabilitation work. We were not sure that Korea was ready for this challenge, but the change in government after the military coup in May, 1961, had given us all new hope for stability and progress. It was upon this hope that we decided to build. The first step in our program would be the training of Korean nationals in administration and in the principles and aims of rehabilitation.

John's proposals were as follows:

(1) Complete reorganization of the Korea amputee rehabilitation project. The program should be limited to the rehabilitation of amputees with the intended purpose of eventually encompassing individuals with other physical disabilities.

(2) Discontinuation of the present vocational training phase of the program, but retention of certain departments such as sewing, woodworking, weaving, handicrafts, which could serve a therapeutic purpose and be supervised by an occupational therapist. This would not be to provide vocational training, but would be an aid in the adjustment of the patient.

(3) Move the project to Seoul, associate it with an ongoing, recognized medical school or large medical center. Prepare blueprints for a new Center in which all departments could be housed in the same building. This would facilitate control and supervision and eliminate the necessity of providing for transport of nonambulatory patients from one section to another.

(4) The proposed program should include the following departments: administration, social service, vocational guidance, prosthetics, physical therapy, occupational therapy. Persons who are best qualified to fill these spots should be sought out. Foreigners now in Korea, with special training in such fields, will be solicited for help and advice in the selection and training of Korean nationals.

(5) Continue to provide academic training or vocational training on a contractual basis with existing Korean facilities. There are a number of these serving the non-handicapped, but experience has shown that they are not averse to training handicapped people also.

(6) Develop an affiliation-training program for students of medicine, social work, and psychology. These areas of social work

and psychology are still weak in Korea and could use the stimulus which a rehabilitation program might offer.

This report, with its sweeping proposals, was submitted in 1961. John followed it with the drastic suggestion that the Taejon Amputee Vocational Training Center be completely closed at the end of the year. Since he had also, with true Dutch prudence, provided a practical way to assure the funds for the building of a new Center in Seoul, the proposal was accepted by Church World Service in New York. Plans for reorganization were under way when we packed up our home and children for a six-month leave at the end of our first term in Korea.

Before leaving the country, we had made arrangements for every amputee on our rolls, disposed of all loose property, completed negotiations with Yonsei University for the location of the new building and submitted the blueprints for it, arranged for the financing of the new Center and for the support of those orphans and student amputees who had been in our care. Those amputees who had received vocational training were helped to find jobs in shops or were provided with the tools of their trade in order to set up in business for themselves. For some the wrench was very difficult. The Center had been their home for years and they had put down roots. When faced with the necessity of self-support, however, most of them proved that they were able to provide for themselves. Only a skeleton staff was maintained, including a limb maker and his helpers who continued to operate a prosthetics shop at Taejon, building new limbs and servicing limbs for students and other indigent amputees during the period that the Center was closed down.

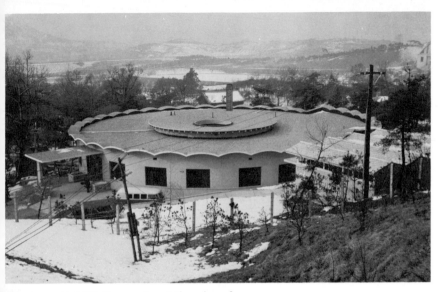

The new rehabilitation center at the edge of
Yonsei University Campus, Seoul.

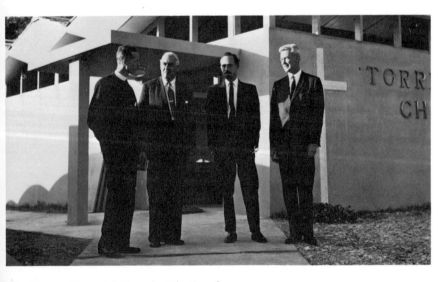

The Torrey Memorial Chapel at the Seoul center.
Left to right: Father Archer Torrey, son of Dr. Torrey;
Leslie Cooke, World Council of Churches; John Steensma;
the late Hugh Farley, Church World Service.

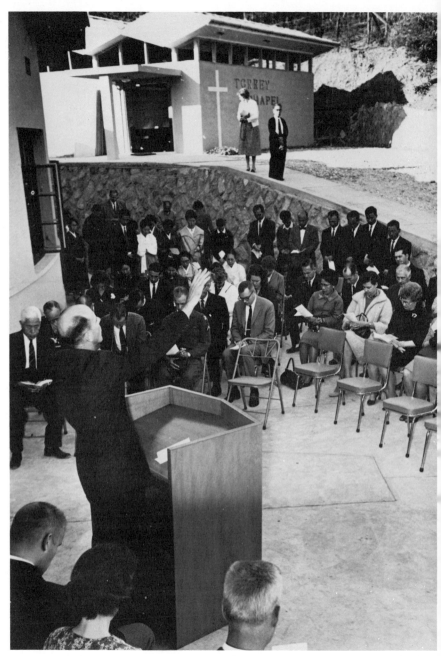
Dr. Samuel Moffett prays at the dedication of the new center.

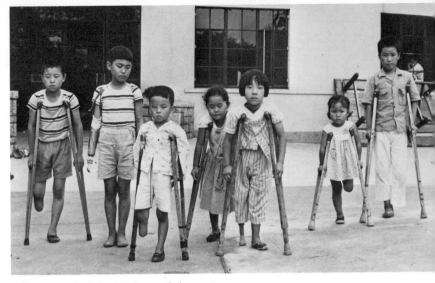

All ages needed the ministry of the center.

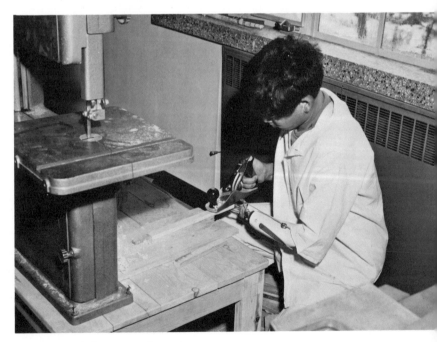

Occupational therapy at the center.

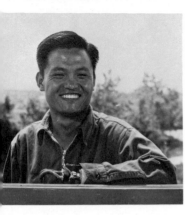

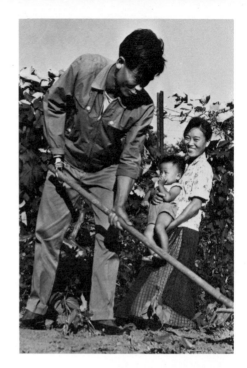

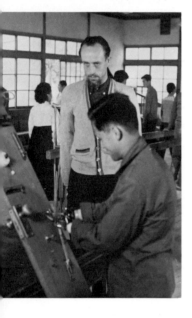

USIS movie,
"With Heart and Hand,"
told the story of
the Taejon center,
using staff and patients
as actors.

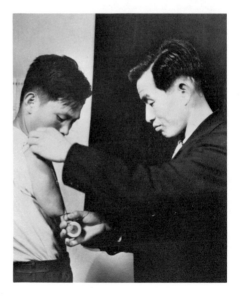

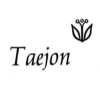

Taejon

9

It was raining heavily when our plane touched down in Seoul at the end of our six months' leave. But it was a different rain than that which had greeted us the first time we landed in Korea. Now we were coming home. Even the rain had a familiar feel as we splashed happily out of the airliner, down the steps onto the puddled concrete. Recognizing beloved friends who were waving and shouting from the observation deck, we called out joyous greetings and hurried inside the terminal building to embrace those dear people whom we had missed so much.

"There's Song *Samonim!*" exclaimed John, as he caught sight of the leg amputee who had been his receptionist, nurse, and clerk at the Taejon amputee center. Mrs. Song was more than a friend. She was indispensable. She could understand John's poor Korean and she refused to make use of an interpreter when she spoke to him. If he failed to understand her, she gestured, explained, sought other words, and persisted in her attempts until he guessed at her meaning. She had an uncanny ability to get the facts out of other amputees who tried to give false information when seeking admittance to the Center. Mrs. Song seemed to have the confidence of everyone; she could see through people yet make them feel as if she would be on their side.

With her, waving a welcome, were her husband, also an amputee, and five children. Four of the children were Songs—the other was another amputee, an orphan whom Mrs. Song had offered to care for after the dormitories at the old Center were closed. We had registered this boy with the Harry Holt Adoption Program in the hope of finding parents in America who might adopt him in spite of his handicap. So far no one had volunteered.

The children immediately picked out Mr. Kim in the waiting crowd. Mr. Kim was our "houseboy," but he had become an important part of the Steensma household. His job combined the duties of a bodyguard, valet, secretary, cook, counselor, friend, and maître d'hotel. For a Korean man, Mr. Kim was larger than average and after many years of carrying the heavy boxes, screwing off tightly-stuck jar lids, and wielding a shovel or a paintbrush myself, a large, strong man around the house was an appreciated addition. Mr. Kim's patient, gentle nature, his willingness, and his loyalty had endeared him to us. He had been the manager of the household. He ordered the food, planned the meals, paid the bills, supervised the work of the other servants. To Mr. Kim, John was always "The Director." He referred to him as "Sir" whether speaking to him or to me about him, and although he was tremendously proud of "Sir" he was also somewhat in awe of him. John did not like to be asked for favors, although he was quick to offer help if he became aware of a real need; so Mr. Kim usually channeled his hints through "Madam." It was then up to "Madam" to head him off when his sensitive feelings were going to be hurt. I would know that although "Sir" would be happy to refer Mr. Kim's wife to the family planning clinic, he was not going to respond politely if Kim asked for relief clothing to give to his housemaid as part of her salary. Mr. Kim was the first to teach us that, to a Korean, there is no shame in presenting a request—whatever it might be. One can ask for anything; the shame falls upon the person who must refuse the request.

Arrangements had been made for us to spend a few days at the Mission Guest House, a comfortable, modestly-priced accomodation for missionaries in transit. There was time to relax there and to rest up after the long trip while the boxes and barrels containing our goods were hauled from the Church World Service warehouse into the house which had been rented for us. This was a huge, three-and-a-half story Western-style structure which stood halfway up the side of a hill on the grounds of Yonsei University and looked grandly down over the little community of Yonhi-dong. As one drove into the city on the airport highway, he could see this house from a distance of three miles.

Perhaps because it was so conspicuously foreign, the house drew the attention of the "slickee boys" in Seoul. Instead of putting bars at the windows, as most householders do in Korea, the owner had rigged up an elaborate electric alarm system. At four o'clock every morning during the first week, this raucous alarm plummeted us out of our beds. The first time it rang, everyone rushed frantically through the house, checking doors and windows to find the broken circuit which might have set off the alarm bell. Nothing seemed disturbed, yet the alarm kept jangling. John gave up in disgust.

"It's a short circuit," he decided. And that was the end of it for him. He flipped off the main switch and went back to bed.

The next morning, the "handyman" (who was furnished with the house) arrived in a state of great excitement. A thief had forced the window of the pumphouse and tried to steal the machinery. The pump was bolted to the concrete upon which it stood, and it was reinforced by cement over the bolts. The would-be-thief had chopped patiently at the cement but had fled when the house lights went on. Unaware that the pumphouse was connected to the alarm system, we had never thought of checking the door and window there.

When the alarm reverberated through the house just before the curfew ended the following night's rest, we knew what to expect. The burglar had come back to finish his work in the pumphouse— this time he was foiled by the outside man who had replaced the chipped cement and reinforced the locks on the door and window.

During the next six months, the reliable alarm and our attractiveness to thieves eliminated any hope of rest. A night's sleep was seldom undisturbed. Whether it was the ostentatious appearance of the place, the lack of bars on the windows, or the knowledge that the occupants of the house were recent arrivals that attracted the night visitors, no one could say. They were persistent enough, trying the windows one by one and once forcing open the lock on the back door. Each time the alarm signaled a new point of entry —a pane of glass removed, a raised window, a cut screen. It was obvious that in time the persevering prowler would discover some way to enter without setting off the bell. The thought of strange, stealthy men wandering through the house, poking and prying about was disturbing. One night I rigged a noisetrap by lining up a row of milk bottles across the entrance from the front hall to the kitchen. When the alarm sent me stumbling sleepily out of a warm bed, an unintentional kick sent the bottles flying across the kitchen linoleum and ricocheting with satisfying crashes. The rest of the family, who had become so used to the ringing of the alarm that it took something special to get them up, flew down the steps to see what was going on. Everyone had a good laugh at Mother, and perhaps even the "slickee boy" was enjoying the party from outside the window.

The only way that anyone could enter this house without tripping the alarm circuit was through a window of the French doors, which opened from the dining room onto the garage roof. These window frames were just large enough so that a small person could squeeze his body through into the room. It could only be a matter of time before this unwanted guest would discover the secret.

A young cousin, who lived with us that year, often sat up late into the night, using the quiet hours to study and to write letters home. One night, about one o'clock, as she sat at one end of the dining table reading a book, she heard tiny, scratching noises.

"It is only the cat," she thought.

Nora had wonderful powers of concentration, but when the small, scraping sounds continued, she forgot her reading and listened intently. Then she heard the unmistakable sound of the opening of the storm door on the patio at her side. She realized immediately that someone had been carefully working loose a pane of glass and now had reached a hand inside and released the lock of the outer door. Next he would try to remove the window glass from the sliding French door. Although Nora was sitting in a lighted room, the draperies drawn across the doors had prevented her from being seen. She quietly left her chair, slipped through the kitchen and up the stairs into the bedroom where we were sleeping.

"Tonight we will catch him," she hissed in my ear. "He's

coming through the French door now! C'mon . . . but be quiet!"

I sneaked downstairs at Nora's heels, my feet bare on the cold floor, my heart pounding with excitement. In the silent house we could hear the clock loudly ticking; the tiny, nicking noises at the window betrayed the presence of the man outside on the garage roof, shivering in the cold as he painstakingly chipped the putty from around the glass. As soon as he had it all out, the action would begin. Whether he poked his head or his feet through the aperture first, a gentle, ladylike tap with Dirk's baseball bat would teach him to stay away from this house in the future.

We stood waiting with bated breath; the moment of truth was at hand. Just then, unaware of our sinister plans, John came into the room. He walked directly to the window and jerked back the traverse drapery. The thief vaulted the balustrade so quickly that we hardly saw him disappear.

It was too much. All my repressed fears came to the surface the next night in a bad nightmare in which I leaped from bed at the sound of the alarm. I struggled with a stranger who was trying to shut it off at the switch box. Then the thief, who had entered the house, came to the stranger's assistance in the fight, while John calmly walked away from us all saying, "You worry too much about it. Just forget it."

The twisting and groaning of the losing fighter finally awakened John and the account of the frightening dream must have convinced him that there is a limit to what a wife can endure. The very next day he petitioned Church World Service for a night guard. The presence of one of the arm amputees, armed with a trusty baseball bat and warmed by a portable kerosene heater as he sat in the back entry, deterred the thieves. They looked for an easier place to rob and the alarm was almost forgotten as night after night passed quietly by.

John's problems were more disturbing, but they bothered him only during the day. There had been an upheaval of staff at Yonsei University, and all of the important personages with whom he had carried on previous negotiations had disappeared. The new people knew nothing of agreements with the amputee rehabilitation center. The plans for construction had been slipped into a file in the

Church World Service office and conveniently forgotten. So John had to begin his planning all over again. He had set up temporary quarters in rented office space and he patiently began the reorganization of his plans to build a new Center. In this effort he was assisted by two faithful retainers who deserve praise for the diligent way in which they had carried on during his absence. Kang Un Tae accurately kept a record of all expenses incurred by our department of Church World Service, and each month he brought in his reliable report to the Seoul office. He maintained a large number of accounts with schools and vocational centers throughout the country where amputees were receiving training. The amputee project continued to subsidize approved hospitals and limb shops where clients could secure care and treatment. Mr. Kang is proof to all doubting foreigners who insist that Koreans cannot be trusted, that a man's nationality or citizenship does not determine his loyalty and honesty.

Kim Young Hyuk, who had served as John's assistant at Taejon, was kept busy completing the survey he was making of amputees who had been helped by the Center, and trying to bring the case histories in our files up-to-date. This experience gave Mr. Kim a new awareness of the nature of rehabilitation and of the need of the disabled for guidance and counsel. He developed a keen interest in social casework, counseling, and the psychology of the handicapped. He often stayed in the office long after closing time to talk with psychiatrists, social workers or patients, or to read a new publication on rehabilitation or counseling.

John had been very upset by the setback in his plans to open the new rehabilitation center in Seoul. As it turned out, the delay gave him opportunity for a careful selection of personnel to staff the various departments in the reorganized program.

One day a young Korean woman walked into the office with greetings and an introduction from Dr. Torrey. She was a social worker, who had just returned to Korea from graduate training at Pendle Hill in Philadelphia. She had very definite ideas of the kind of work she was looking for and she was not sure that the amputee rehabilitation project met her specifications. John was intrigued. Usually, when applicants came looking for a job, they presented their credentials and then waited for *his* approval. Oh Chang Hie was the type of person who knew exactly what she wanted. She had an air of refinement, was tastefully dressed and completely poised, and she spoke flawless English. More amazing, she could drive a car—an unusual accomplishment for a Korean lady!

She informed him sweetly that she would like to find out more about the work of the rehabilitation center among the Korean people. She was not interested in a job with prestige or with a high salary. All she asked was the opportunity to use her education and abilities to help her own people directly. Needless to say, John and Kim Young Hyuk were impressed and waited anxiously while Miss Oh made inquiries about the amputee project. They hoped that she would decide to join it, for they recognized that she would be an exceptional and valuable addition to the staff.

Miss Oh became a tremendous asset to the rehabilitation center. From the day she joined it until she left, to be with her husband who was a doctor in America, she was the backbone of the social work program. She had the gift of being at ease with anyone, and whether she sat at dinner with ambassadors and prime ministers or crouched on the floor of the meanest hut, she was able to adapt herself to her surroundings and to charm those around her. Her tact and her gracious manner never failed. It is to Oh Chang Hie that the work of rehabilitation owes much of its success.

The discussions with Yonsei University over a suitable site dragged on. Finally a location directly behind the new Severance Hospital, between Church World Service Crippled Children's Center and the tomb of a deceased Korean queen, was offered for the amputee rehabilitation center. The location bordered the medical school and the nursing college of Yonsei University and was also very close to the great women's college of Korea, Ewha University. Since Ewha had a school of social work, this would be an ideal beginning for the program which John had planned—to make the amputee center also a supervised training center for social work students.

The frustrations faced in trying to build a new rehabilitation center would have deterred a less stubborn man than John Steensma. He had become accustomed to government red tape, but when he was informed that the site selected by Yonsei University was part of a national treasure because of its proximity to the tomb of a dead queen, he almost gave up. Still, it was only a small corner of the cultural monument and there was hope that the government might be convinced that the need of live cripples spoke louder than the honor of a departed queen. When permission was finally granted to Yonsei University to use the land, it was discovered that the university had made a mistake in surveying it. All the documents came back to be done over again; one by one they had to be presented at the proper offices, sealed with the proper seals, bought with the stated price.

At last the building permit was granted and ground was broken for the new amputee rehabilitation center in the spring of 1963, one year and four months after the Taejon Amputee Vocational Center had closed down.

🌷10

A whole year had passed. Perhaps the year had not really been lost, however. Amputees who had looked forward to presenting themselves at the old shelter had been forced to find a new haven. Staff members who had previously run the vocational training shops had established themselves by this time in businesses of their own and not only earned a living but were hiring other amputees in their shops. The staff members had had the opportunity to increase their knowledge of sound social casework and rehabilitation practice. John was cautious in employing staff, although there had been no decrease in the number of new cases that presented themselves at the weekly clinics. Social casework was in its infancy in Korea, and each new caseworker required individual instruction and supervision. He had used the time of waiting to meet those missionaries and other people in Seoul who could be of service in the establishment of a solid program of social welfare and total rehabilitation. Members of the Yonsei Medical School assured him of their cooperation and participation, and he began to look forward with anticipation toward the day when educational, medical, and rehabilitative facilities would be fruitfully coordinated to serve the handicapped people of Korea.

As soon as the Center received a building permit, the site became a beehive of activity. Cement mixers began to churn, the bricks began to rise in rows, and the Korea Amputee Rehabilitation Center began to take shape. It was a strange shape in Korea—a circular building which lay among the trees like a huge doughnut when one looked down on it from the crest of the hill. On the outer ring of the doughnut were the offices of the receptionist, accountant, and director; an occupational therapy room; a physical therapy room; the limb shop with fitting booths; men's and women's dormitories and baths; the front and rear entrance lobbies and a warehouse. On the inner circle were the offices of four social workers, the kitchen and dining room and a laundry-lavatory. Construction proceeded rapidly and without serious setbacks. The contractor was cooperative and soon our satisfaction in the appearance of the building and in the quality of the work had exceeded everyone's expectation.

When summer came, our fifteen-year-old son expressed a desire to earn some money of his own and the contractor at the building site offered him a job on his construction crew. Perhaps Dirk thought that as the son of the director he would receive special treatment. He might have expected favoritism because he was a foreigner. His five years' experience in Korea had been somewhat sheltered and his only knowledge of the life of the average Korean laborer was based on the casual observation and limited understanding of an American schoolboy.

The contractor, Mr. Lee, liked Dirk. He encouraged him at his new job, but since he was a fair man he also warned Dirk that he would have to start at the bottom and keep up with the other workers. Dirk was eager and determined to succeed. He felt that he had to prove to Mr. Lee, to his parents, and especially to the young Koreans who worked for Lee that an American boy could pull his own weight. With the broiling sun on his back and the perspiration dripping off his nose, Dirk sat for hours chipping concrete off used bricks. It was a humble job and it blistered his hands, but he did not quit. Soon the Korean boys of his age began to offer friendship, stopping by to chat and eat their lunch with him. In a few weeks, Dirk was promoted to the next job up the scale and he was as proud as if he had graduated. (And so were his parents!) His muscles toughened and he began to find pleasure in his work. He appreciated the money which he had earned by his own sweat, but he was more impressed by the firsthand knowledge of what it means to earn a living on the Korean economy. This experience taught him respect and sympathy for the day laborer who has to work so hard to earn so little.

The English language newspaper in Seoul needed a copyreader and English consultant, so John suggested that I keep myself busy there until the amputee program could move into the new building and resume its normal operation. Although this job offered plenty of opportunity to make a contribution, there was far more for a foreign staff member to learn than to teach. Living in the country for three years, surrounded by the placid beauty of the landscape, I had become accustomed to the gentle courage of the people and the dignity and simplicity of their way of life. The city, especially here in company of the sophisticated, highly-educated young journalists, showed a different aspect of Korea—this was a Korea which was eager to take its place in the world, a Korea which resented being represented as a beggar. I was introduced to the power at the top—the political intrigues in the capital, the scandals in government and business, the manipulations which went on behind the headlines. The lessons taught by these intelligent young co-workers changed and enlarged my view of Korea. Seoul is a teeming city— every bit as interesting, but entirely different from the "land of the morning calm" which one finds in the country areas. The *Korea Times* reporters held a wet finger to the wind—a shooting incident on the DMZ, a fight in the National Assembly, a plane crash, an election. Excitement built up quickly in the office as the reporters and editors gathered around the telephone and passed the news from desk to desk.

A disadvantage in this situation was due partly to the fact that I had never learned to speak Korean language fluently. Everyone at *Korea Times* worked in the English language. The men were very polite and they conversed with each other in English when I was included; but when a scoop came in and tension mounted, they naturally began to shout at each other in Korean. Just when events became the most exciting, I was least able to follow them.

There was also a disadvantage in being a woman. The Korean woman has her own place and both she and her menfolk understand what it is. Neither the Korean men in the office nor I was quite sure of the place of a foreign woman. The natural courtesy of the Koreans must have suffered its greatest strain at this point, and my American feminist training also groaned a bit. Sometimes I seethed with insignificance when a guest came into the office and was politely introduced to everyone else while I was completely ignored. But a degree of the humility and modesty proper to women in Korea eventually became practical in this world of Korean men, and in time we came to an understanding of each other.

Gradually, my new friends at the *Times* began to express themselves and their opinions as we talked together. Early in our acquaintance, I had identified myself as a Christian. No one was particularly surprised or impressed by this, but they wondered why I wanted to be called a "missionary." Some of the reporters had met John and were familiar with his work and his affiliation with Church World Service, and they did not consider this a missionary organization. In their minds, as in the minds of many American people, a "missionary" is an evangelist. Further discussion on the subject revealed that the image of the missionary in Korea has become somewhat tarnished during the postwar years. Contempt was openly expressed for some prominent missionaries who had used their personal reputation or the power and money of their supporting organization to manipulate Koreans. We reached an agreement that there are some Christian missionaries who still sacrifice and who are spending themselves for the good of the Korean people, but admitted that missionaries are human beings and there are some who patronize Koreans and who constantly present Korea to the Western world as a beaten nation, poor and dirty. There are some who, like other human beings, have rather obvious failings; some who are ineffectual or lazy; some who are saints.

These Korean men at the *Times* office were sure of themselves, they were proud of their country and of its history, they were willing to work for its future. Our afternoon breaks in the tearoom often turned into lively discussion periods and gave me a wide base from which to view Korea.

The newspaper also opened up new doors for rehabilitation. Both John and I were permitted to use a daily column to present the problems of the disabled to the Korean public. Since the paper used English, it was read only by foreigners and by Korean students and educated people—the very portion of the population we were trying to reach. The column also opened up other interesting outlets—invitations to teach English, assignments to write articles for other papers, a request to write a book of English conversation for Korean students. We met many new friends through this contact —people wrote to the amputee center to find help in their difficulties, some hoped to acquire an American pen pal, others wanted money or sponsorship to America. Some were post-polio cripples and begged for a miracle. Others only wanted to argue. I answered them all.

Working with Korean English was either exasperating or hilarious. Teachers of English in Korean schools stress vocabulary, and a Korean writer can use words which the average American reader has never seen in print. He strains to make a place for his new words, and the results are often too obvious. The sentences become stiff and unwieldy and sometimes the meaning is entirely buried under a tangle of words. One must handle such a paragraph like a tangled ball of yarn. Each thread of thought must be carefully worked out and separated, and sometimes the whole thing is so knotted that it is necessary to throw it out and begin all over again.

Some of the errors were so amusing that I carried them home to share with the family. This always meant an English lesson for Mr. Kim. Kim had previously been employed as a cook for the United States Army and although he had learned to speak English, he was quick to appreciate the difference between the kind of language we spoke in our home and the kind he had heard in the barracks. Sometimes he slipped and called a "spade" a "shovel" and then he was miserable in his chagrin. We cooperated with his frank request to correct him and teach him "good English," and the lessons continued for the entire eight years that Mr. Kim worked for us. It seemed to be a worthwhile endeavor, since Mr. Kim had learned Chinese characters in high school and could already read, write, and speak some Japanese as well as English. The progress he made in English would insure him of a steady job with a foreign organization after we left Korea.

Some of the best jokes at the *Korea Times* were never printed. When the wife of the Korean President visited the various hospitals and prisons and brought each inmate a little package containing soap, toothpaste, and other small items to add to his comfort, a cub reporter featured the excursion in a headline which proclaimed: "PRESIDENT'S WIFE MAKES COMFORT STOP." This was almost too cute to resist sharing with American readers who would discover the nugget at their breakfast tables and chuckle over it all day at their desks. Loyalty to the *Korea Times* was stronger than temptation and I regretfully rewrote the headline. But the story about the girl who worked her way through college by delivering the morning newspaper slipped through as it was written and everyone shared the joke in the caption: "MISS LEE HAS DIFFICULT TIME IN DELIVERY."

The work at the *Korea Times* never became boring, but the problem of getting back and forth from the office through the busy traffic of Seoul finally defeated me. On lucky days the vehicle from the Center would be waiting at the door at quitting time. Otherwise there were three choices: I could walk, ride a taxi, or a taxi-bus.

On fair days walking was enjoyable exercise after an afternoon of sitting in the drab, sooty *Times* office. It afforded a wonderful opportunity to see, hear, and smell life on the Korean streets.

Taxis were not expensive, if you were familiar with the going rate, but they were not always available for a long ride during the busy hours.

The "hapsung" (a combination taxi-bus) offered as much in the way of diversion as a walk, and cost about four cents for the four-mile ride to our part of the city. "Hapsung" were dangerously exciting. On a tight schedule, the little buses careened into the curbstop, barely pausing long enough for passengers to leap into them. The comfort and safety of those who rode was a secondary consideration of the cowboy who drove, and passengers were packed in and shaken up without any thought.

Although Seoul is full of foreigners these days, a foreigner does not go unnoticed in the "hapsung." His very presence there identifies him as one who enjoys association with Korean people. The foreign rider is often treated as a guest. A Korean might graciously offer his seat or the bus girl might forget to ask for his fare. Children stared at the stranger with shyness or curiosity and students always grasped the chance to practice their English conversation. It followed a predictable pattern:

"Excuse me, please. I am Korean student." This was obvious, since they all wear a school uniform with the name of the school pinned to the breast pocket. So I merely smiled and nodded and replied, "Hello."

"I should like to speak English with you."

Another smile, another nod. "All right."

"May I ask you a question?" There would follow a long, painful pause while the questioner considered his question. At last he would blurt out, *"How old are you?"* This offered the opportunity to direct the conversation out of the rut by telling him that American women hate to be asked their age, but sometimes it was simpler just to tell him how old I was and wait for the next question from page one of the paperback English conversation book which every young Korean person seems to carry in his pocket.

There were buses in Seoul too, but during the rush hour they demanded more longanimity than I had yet developed. Bodies were packed in tightly and hanging out over the step. People elbowed each other's ribs and stamped on each other's toes. They carried on all sorts of bundles—babies and bottles of cooking oil, even livestock. They carried off all sorts of goods too—wristwatches were nimbly cut from extended arms and purses were severed from the straps still tightly clutched by owners who were struggling to keep their balance in the swaying, lurching vehicle. Even the tightly-compressed bodies did not heat the interior of the buses in the winter and in warm weather the odors defied all attempts at ventilation.

A ride through the streets of Seoul was never dull. One could expect to see all sorts of goods displayed in the open stalls—fruits and vegetables piled in colorful pyramids, bright tubs of red peppers like traffic lights among the pots of salt and rice, the rubber shoes for ladies in a pastel rainbow across the front of a store, and the red, blue, and green shoes of the children. Displays of art work, racks of ready-to-wear, gleaming white porcelain toilets proudly displayed in front of the shops—all flashed past the windows of the speeding "hapsung." In the streets, the rich brocades of the women contrasted sharply with the neat, dark uniforms of the students. Toddlers with round little bottoms shining bare in their open-crotched pants, squatted on the sidewalks, and beggars with matted hair peered out of their dirty rags as they hunched on the curbs. Sometimes one would see a mentally deranged person running half naked down the center of the road, laughing and screaming hysterically. Even the signs were unusual. Many of them attempted English, often with ludicrous results. We became accustomed to the invitation to "RUBRICATION" but everyone remained dubious about the sign downtown which stated: "MAY PARKING HERE."

All the sights were not pleasant. Traffic accidents were so frequent that more than once I have seen children mangled in the street by a heedless truck or bus. The cruel mistreatment of dumb animals and the miseries of human beings who had to live like animals was painful to watch. Seoul is an honest city, and anyone who rides through her streets with open eyes must see her as she is.

Sometimes there was a surprise waiting at home. Often it would be an unexpected but welcomed guest—a soldier from a nearby camp, a missionary from one of the more distant stations, or a friend who was passing near and decided to drop in for tea. Mr. Kim was a hospitable stand-in host. He invited every foreigner to come in and offered him coffee or a cold drink as he rested in the living room. With his own people he was more selective, having learned by experience that Korean visitors come for many reasons and sometimes they are harder to get out than in.

One day Mr. Kim ran outside to meet me as I walked up the drive. Although he was so flustered that he forgot to remove his apron, he greeted me with a forced calm and a shocking announcement.

"Madam," he said. "There is a dead woman in our garden."

"Really, Mr. Kim? Have you seen her yourself?" If there was really a corpse in our garden, Mr. Kim would steer clear of it. He was careful about getting involved with anything that he couldn't handle.

"See for yourself," he shrugged, and disappeared into the house to watch gleefully from the window. He had pointed out a copse of trees at the far edge of the garden so I walked over to look. There, in the midst of the trees, someone had dug a shallow grave. In it lay what could have been a small body, uncovered, but wrapped in rice-straw mats. A pair of boat-shaped, white rubber shoes stood neatly together at the edge of the hole and a big bundle wrapped with a towel lay a little to one side. Between the mats, a head of coarse black Korean hair left no doubt that this was indeed a body.

Mr. Kim did not miss my shock, but my first question shook him out of his smugness. "Don't you think we should call the police?"

"Oh, no!" protested my cook. "They will bother us for a long time and interrupt our work all week." As a rule, Korean citizens have no wish to become involved with the police. They do not yet think of the police force as a protective and helpful organization. Mr. Kim had already solved this problem in his own way by spreading the news of his discovery to a few neighboring villagers. The affair was soon out of our hands. A crowd was converging at the site and a police jeep drove up the road at the bottom of the hill. The body was quickly removed and the area roped off. Mr. Kim went down into the crowd to pick up the gossip and reported that the police suspected a hit-and-run driver who had panicked and tried to hide the body of his victim. Who he was or who the dead lady was is still a mystery. It is even difficult to make some of our friends believe that the corpse was in our garden at all. They suspect it was just another nightmare.

11

*B*efore going to America to study, Miss Oh had worked among the refugees who lived in the shacks along the banks of the Han River. She knew the area well and when she invited me to accompany her on home visits one day, I accepted gladly. She herself drove the new Land Rover which had just arrived as a gift from the Oxford Famine Relief Committee. The vehicle jogged through the hardened ruts and bounced over the stones of alleyways as we squeezed between the ramshackle buildings in search of the room which a family of three called home. Inside the five-foot square cubbyhole lay a hunchbacked man with his crutches on the floor beside him. He looked weak and sick, but when he recognized Miss Oh he smiled a welcome. Obviously she was an old friend.

No, he was not much better, he told her. Things were very difficult for the family. It was not the amputation, but the lung disease that kept him down. A spasm of coughing interrupted the conversation and the man lay back exhausted.

Outside, his wife was cooking something over a little fire. Even though it was a cold January day, she did all her cooking outside because there was no kitchen. Things were going from bad to worse, she said, and she didn't think she could stand it much longer.

Miss Oh was silent in sympathy. The wife called out to her little daughter, who was playing nearby with a group of other children. When the child caught sight of the visitor, she ran toward us joyfully. Miss Oh embraced her and inquired about her school, her friends, and her activities. The little girl thanked her for the clothes that she had brought on her last visit, and Miss Oh promised that next time she came she would bring a treat. Then the mother confided that she often thinks of taking the child with her and leaving her husband. Trying to care for him and earn enough to feed them all is too difficult, she said.

I felt quite inadequate in the face of such need. My impulse was to offer food and clothing at once. But Miss Oh, who was wiser and more understanding, sensed that this woman needed comfort and reassurance so she chatted easily with her for a few minutes, petting and praising the little girl and encouraging the mother. Then, promising to return soon, she said good-bye. Later, she discussed the case at the staff meeting of social workers and proposed that we help the mother to set up a small business in her home. In this way she could take care of her husband while she earned enough money to keep the family together.

The next house was not so hard to find. It was one of the nicest in the neighborhood. We were graciously invited to come in and sit on the warm floor to have refreshments. The foreign guest was ushered to the place of honor—the hottest spot on the floor. At first it felt wonderful for my cold toes, but it did not take long before my manners became strained by the discomfort of the honorable position, and I began a series of surreptitious shifts to avoid the warmth of hospitality underneath.

The front of the house contained a tiny grocery store, and the family grandmother hurriedly filled a tray from its shelves and presented us an offering of crackers and candies. Miss Oh, taking no chances with my American appetite or my lack of exposure to a tight economy, warned me in rapid English that the contents of the tray would make an appreciable difference in the margin of profit for the day. While we nibbled politely and chatted with our hostess, four dirty little children poked their black faces around the sliding door at the rear. Their mother apologized for their appearance, explaining that they played in the coal which the family stored and sold in the community. The father, a leg amputee, was off on his bicycle, peddling goods. Miss Oh seemed pleased by the industry and progress which this family evidenced and she told me that when the father had first appeared at the rehabilitation center for help, they had been on the edge of starvation.

After leaving this friendly home, we drove to a camp for flood victims. The houses were pieced together from slats of board, scraps of tin, and bits of canvas. Miss Oh parked the Rover alongside a dwelling which had been temporarily constructed by piling cement blocks upon one another and stretching a canvas across the top. Here we found another amputee father with his wife and five young children. When he had come to the center clinic, said Miss Oh, he was a beggar and could barely keep his family alive by the trade. The mother and her youngest child had been sick and the father was desperate. After being fitted with a new leg and given training in walking with it, the man was given a few chickens so that he could earn some income. The chickens prospered, and now the family sold the eggs. It was only a little, but Miss Oh pointed out that it was very important for rehabilitation workers to share the burden which this father carried if they really wanted to help him to lead a productive life. Now that he had made a beginning, she had faith that he would really try to stand on his own feet again and support his own family.

Before going back to the amputee center, we stopped in to see Oh Dok Hwan. Mr. Oh was an old acquaintance who had a long history of refractory behavior, but having known him at his worst, we appreciated his evident rehabilitation. He was in the garden at the Anglican Seminary wielding a rake with one hand and his hook prosthesis when we saw him, but as soon as he recognized the Rover he dropped his rake and ran toward it. A wide smile lighting up his face, Mr. Oh proudly introduced us to a beaming young woman who held a fat, naked baby.

"Here is my wife. This is my son." Oh Dok Hwan was showing off his ability in English language for my benefit and for the benefit of his friends and neighbors who were gathering around us. Then, switching to his own language, he explained to them who we were. Even though Miss Oh was a much more important member of the rehabilitation team than I, to Mr. Oh and his village friends the visit from the wife of the foreign director seemed to represent some sort of extra in prestige value.

Over a long period of association, Oh Dok Hwan's history had become quite familiar to us. When his father was drafted to forced labor in Japan, the mother ran off with another man and her pampered little son continued to be indulged. But when the father returned, he seized the child and spirited him South across the 38th parallel. Times were hard in those days, especially for refugees, and the boy not only became separated from his father but was forced to beg for his food. Finally he heard that his father had been killed. He became an aimless wanderer then, hanging around the American Army camps and currying favor with GIs. When a mine explosion tore off his arm, he was put into an Army hospital. Eventually, he landed in an orphanage.

Making use of the same charm and warm smile which had stood him in good stead with the Americans, Oh soon became a favorite of the orphanage director. In the orphanage he also made friends with a girl, and the two of them grew up together. When they became old enough, Oh asked permission of the superintendent to marry the girl. The reaction was one of shock and dismay. The superintendent was a devout Christian and he had entertained dreams of this young man as a leader in the church. He saw Oh's relationship to a girl only as sinful lust. Oh Dok Hwan was given a stern lecture, separated from his friend, and enrolled in a boarding school for boys.

Perhaps at this stage an experienced social worker could have helped Mr. Oh, but there were no social workers in Korea then. The guardians decided that the boy needed sterner discipline. Instead of being pampered, his freedom was curtailed and he was closely watched. He learned to lie and he became clever at sneaking out to see his girl at the orphanage. When he was expelled from the school in disgrace, the American missionary who had been contributing toward his support suggested that he be sent to the Taejon Vocational Training Center for amputees. It seemed a good way to get rid of Oh Dok Hwan.

Of course he did not tell us of his escapades when he requested admittance. He looked like an amiable and bright young man, and we needed an amiable and bright young man as gardener and handyman at our house. Working around an American home kept Oh interested for a little while, but he could not resist prying into drawers, inspecting our personal possessions, and eavesdropping on conversations. Our annoyance and Mr. Oh's restlessness soon separated us. By this time, Mr. Oh had had enough of interference with his life and he cut himself loose from the supervision of the amputee center. With a companion who was a heavy drinker, he began to hang around the wine shops in the city. The two amputees used their hooks to threaten the townspeople and to force money from them. In this way they supported themselves and stayed drunk.

The first time these wild young men visited the amputee center, they simply made a nuisance of themselves. The director refused to be intimidated and warned them sternly to stay away. This made Oh furious. He returned with his companion one night and terrorized everyone with his drunken brawling and vandalism. Mr. Oh was apprehended by the police, identified as the culprit, and put into jail.

He had been living with his girl friend from the orphanage, and while he served his prison sentence she gave birth to a baby. Mr. Oh loved this girl and worried about her and his son. He resolved to change his life when he was released from prison and do his best to support the girl and his baby. Affairs were not that simple, however. Oh Dok Hwan's intentions were strong, but his reputation was even stronger. He found all doors closed to him. Mr. Oh's case is an illustration of the failure of the Taejon amputee center to deal with the emotional and social problems which often accompanied an amputee's physical disability. When Mr. Oh was living at the Center, there had been no attempt to understand the background causes of a client's antisocial behavior. He had simply been dismissed because of his refusal to cooperate.

Mr. Oh did not give up, however. Reduced once again to begging, he sent a letter to the rehabilitation center in Seoul with a plea to reconsider his need. When he was called in for counseling, he explained his new motivation and he confessed that he still had a problem with his drinking. It was evident that many of his old hostilities still troubled him, yet he seemed eager to discuss them and eliminate them. He was referred to the Korean psychiatrist at the Yonsei Medical Center. In the meantime, Father Archer Torrey, who maintained an active interest in the work which his father had begun, offered to give Mr. Oh another chance and to accept him as an apprentice on the Anglican Mission farm project. In consultation with the psychiatrist, Mr. Oh began to realize that many of his problems were the result of childhood insecurity and forced submissiveness. His resentments had been repressed until they had finally found expression under the influence of alcohol. His love for his childhood sweetheart was real and lasting, but it had been dismissed by his guardians as a passing fancy. Mr. Oh asked permission to bring his common-law wife and his son to Seoul with him to live at the farm, and Father Torrey suggested a Christian marriage ceremony for them.

"How is everything going now?" asked the social worker, and Oh Dok Hwan confidently bobbed his head at her. "Good! Good!" he replied.

"No problems?" probed Miss Oh. She had heard that sometimes Mr. Oh still gets drunk. But he has become a steady worker, a faithful husband, and a good neighbor. His neighbors liked him and accepted him. He himself has accepted his handicap, admitted his weaknesses, and recognized that the social worker, the priest, and the psychiatrist are his friends. Their help has been as necessary to Oh Dok Hwan as the help of the limb maker.

Those of us who had worked at the rehabilitation center had assumed, as a matter of course, that the difficulties which the disabled people of Korea experienced were due solely to the prejudice of society. Korea, we stated, represented a culture which placed no value upon human dignity and considered a handicapped person totally without value. We could support this theory by examples. Consider the case of the amputee woman who earned her living by bearing children to her employers. When a man's wife failed to conceive, this woman was "hired" for a year or two. During this time she was expected to become pregnant and to give birth to a living child. As soon as this occurred, the infant was snatched from the mother and became the child of her employer and his wife. When she came to the rehabilitation center, the woman had borne three children to three different men. The Korean people would probably consider such a woman not as a person at all, but more as an incubator. We would surmise that such an abuse of human dignity was the result of her amputation. But as we lived longer among the Korean people and became more and more familiar with the backgrounds and attitudes of those who came to the rehabilitation center for help, we gradually revised our opinions about social prejudice.

John explained it to the social workers this way: "When I go out among American people," he said, "I am often introduced to a new acquaintance. The natural gesture of an American who meets another for the first time is to shake hands. So I extend my hook in place of a hand. To a person who has never seen a prosthetic appliance, this is a shocking surprise. If he is poised and self-possessed, he may grasp it with only momentary hesitation. But some people react with embarrassment and quickly withdraw an extended hand."

"That is not prejudice!" objected one of the social workers.

"No," answered John. "It is neither prejudice nor rejection. It is unfamiliarity, possibly—or simply embarrassment. But how can I know that? If I were sensitive about my own lack of ability to shake hands, couldn't I interpret this withdrawal as rejection on the part of others?"

John had a point. If the amputees could learn to accept themselves, others might accept them too. If a person is convinced of his own worth, will he allow others to treat him as subhuman? Had we been approaching the whole problem backwards, working to educate the public when we should have been working first of all with the amputee himself and his attitude? In a society which waged a constant struggle against unemployment and overpopulation, there would never be enough room for the weak and defeated. Therefore, we must help our amputees to believe in themselves in order to give them strength and self-assurance.

Kim Young Hyuk called this program the "Freedom from Prejudice Movement" and he dedicated himself to its advancement. He organized a club with thirty handicapped members and thirty-five non-handicapped members in the Seoul area. Each month this club sponsored a social gathering, inviting both handicapped and non-handicapped guests in the hope that by getting to know each other they could eliminate the uneasiness that might cause prejudice between them. We were happy to see this initiative on the part of Mr. Kim and the response of the Korean people, especially the young people, to it. The Freedom from Prejudice movement seemed to be off to a good start in building bridges of understanding between society and the disabled.

12

According to the plaque, hung in the entrance lobby, the Korea Church World Service Rehabilitation Center was dedicated to the glory of God and to the welfare of the handicapped people of Korea on October 31, 1963. Friends, colleagues, patients, staff members, and representatives of supporting organizations gathered for the dedication ceremony of the new building.

To most of those who gathered with us, it was probably only another function among the many which they had attended that year. "Command performances" were a price one had to pay when one lived in Seoul, and our schedule, like that of everyone else, was filled with teas, receptions, dedications, commemorations, and honorary presentations which we attended dutifully. To John and to me, to the staff members and patients of the amputee center, this day marked more than the dedication of a building. We were dedicating ourselves and our service to God. His blessing and his guidance in the development of the rehabilitation center up to this point had been clear to us all and we acknowledged it with thanksgiving. All of us were very much aware of the tremendous task we had assumed and of our dependence upon God's help for the success of this work.

Our hearts joined in the words of the soloist as she sang:

Thine arm, O Lord, in days of old
Was strong to heal and save;

It triumphed o'er disease and death,
O'er darkness and the grave.
To Thee they went, the blind, the dumb,
The palsied and the lame,
The leper with his tainted life,
The sick with fevered frame.

Be Thou our great Deliverer still,
Thou Lord of life and death;
Restore and quicken, soothe and bless
With Thine almighty breath.
To hands that work and eyes that see,
Give wisdom's heavenly lore,
That whole and sick, and weak and strong,
May praise Thee evermore.

Adjoining the rehabilitation center was a separate chapel, named in honor of the founder of the rehabilitation work in Korea. "Torrey Chapel" was the contribution of Christian friends in America and in Korea. Although Church World Service did not feel that the chapel program was a legitimate part of rehabilitation service and would not include it in the annual budget or in the estimated cost of the new building, we were convinced that the religious emphasis was the foundation of the entire project and could not be eliminated. A whole man includes both body and soul. We had come to Korea to witness to the love and mercy of Christ, and although we made no effort to evangelize, we believed that the ministry of our chaplain, public worship by those of us who confessed the name of Christ, and a religious program for all who might be interested or curious was essential. The funds for the erection and furnishing of the chapel and for the ongoing chapel program were donated as special gifts by others who believed as we did, and permission was given by Yonsei University and by Church World Service to construct the chapel building next to the Center.

This chapel was in use every day of the week. Besides two Sunday services, Sunday school for the neighborhood children, and a midweek prayer service on Wednesday, it was used as a school-room for children whose parents were unable to afford the public schools. This was a volunteer effort by our staff members. They canvassed the area around the Center and invited the children to the school. The immediate response was overwhelming, so only those who were most needy were allowed to remain. Out of their own salaries, the volunteer teachers bought classroom supplies. School hours began after offices closed at the amputee center. Each evening, around four-thirty, the children began to arrive at the gate. By five they were clamoring to enter. They ran to their classroom with joy—and I watched with amazement for it had been a long time since I had seen children so eager for school.

Since these children represented homes which were so poor that the parents could not afford to pay for school supplies or fees or the required school uniform, and because there was no law in Korea which requires the attendance of children at public school, these youngsters were doomed to grow up as illiterates. It was not only for this reason that we were happy with the volunteer school in the amputee center. It was evidence that the Korean people were not content merely to accept help which American churches had sent to them in their need. These rehabilitation workers, who had shared the joy of people who once thought of themselves as useless and now had been given an opportunity to make a contribution with their lives, had learned the blessing of service and were trying to pass it on to their neighbors.

We were proud of our new quarters. The unusual round building contained dormitory space for thirty-five patients. They slept, Korean-style, on pads laid on the floor, but they used chairs in the dining room because it is difficult for leg amputees to sit down and get up again off the floor. John, who insisted on the standards of cleanliness taught by his Dutch mother, made regular inspections of the kitchen, bathrooms, and dormitories. His prying eye was everywhere. Every limb made in the limb shop was checked at the weekly clinics for workmanship, fit, alignment, appearance; and every patient was given the chance to voice his opinions. John helped to prepare the menus, using the donated Church World Service foods wherever possible. With Mr. Kang, he worked out the budget to be presented to the main office of CWS; with Kim Young Hyuk, he made decisions concerning present and future policy; he attended the regular meetings of the social workers at which they discussed their cases together and approved the nurse's decisions to refer patients for medical treatment. He was delighted when the Korean staff vetoed his suggestion to give a patient money or relief clothing. "Americans give too easily," they told him. "Let us handle it."

No new patients were admitted during the first few months in the new building while we checked the records of cases already on the files, visited homes and schools of all sponsored amputee students, and wrote individual reports to all their sponsors. We also tried to broaden the scope and experience of the staff members by inviting guest speakers to instruct them on subjects such as family planning and social work. Lively discussions over the role of the psychiatrist in rehabilitation or the cause and prevention of parasites in the Korean population were stimulated by films. John realized that if he hoped to hand over the responsibility for rehabilitation to the Korean workers, he must prepare them. He must also give them an idea of the professional services that were available to help them.

At the beginning of 1964, we were ready to open the doors of the rehabilitation center to new patients. John stressed a quality approach, adding gradually to the patient load as the staff increased and became capable of handling more people. It was clear at once to me, as well as to John, that running a hospital-center was going to be hard work. Details and decisions, more details and more decisions filled the first few days. As a starter, ten patients were admitted; before they arrived we had to organize the cooks and plan the meals, buy the furniture for the dining room and the pots and pans and cups and bowls and chopsticks for the kitchen. The huge pressure cooker in which food for the patients would be prepared must have a practice run. The volatile contraption frightened us nearly as much as it did the Korean cooks!

Someone was sent to pick up a bale of bedding from the Church World Service warehouse; someone else was assigned the duty of washing enough blankets for incoming patients; pillows and sheets had to be quickly prepared; charts were run off the duplicating machine—with constant interruptions by telephone or by people who stopped in "for just a look"—and all the while we must not get behind on correspondence, clinics, lectures, staff meetings, shopping, limb making, report writing, or guest tours.

I became John's amanuensis while he drove off in all directions. The nurse came running in to announce that one of our new patients had brought his own lice with him. "Wash everything over again!" I ordered. "All the bedding, all the clothes. And next time, wash the patient *first!*"

We made fifty pairs of pajamas, and each new arrival was stripped of his clothing for laundering. But we had forgotten to make underwear . . . and underwear was absolutely necessary to the modesty of a patient who was constantly asked to exhibit his artificial limb and the straps which controlled it.

Patients were referred to the Center in various ways. Some read of it in the newspapers or heard of the service from others. Many amputees were brought in by missionaries or by Korean pastors. Each new patient was initially interviewed by a Korean social worker before he was admitted, and records were kept in both the Korean and the English languages. This interview established a relationship between the caseworker and the patient. Naturally, we could not always depend upon this information. One boy of eleven years, when admitted to the Center, told the caseworker a touching story of being separated from his parents in some accident when he was five years old. He described in a very convincing manner how he had roamed the streets, begging for his food. The caseworker did not question the story, but set about making friends with the little boy. As they began to know each other, the child talked about his relatives in the South. Without any fuss, the social worker journeyed to the area he had mentioned to investigate this lead . . . but found nothing. When she reported her failure, the boy was upset by the needless expense and effort. He confessed that he had lied to her.

"I really do know where my parents are," he admitted. "My brother lives with them—and my little sister too." His home, he said, was above the 38th parallel in the Demilitarized Zone.

When the social worker visited the family, they were happy to hear that the boy was alive and well, but showed no anxiety about getting him back. It would mean feeding another mouth, and the father barely managed to earn enough for his wife and the two remaining children.

"We thank you for caring for our son," the father said politely. "Nobody knew where he had gone, and he is my eldest son. Is it possible that you would keep him?"

The social worker explained that it would be impossible. She praised the lad's intelligence and the quick way in which he had gained skills with the artificial arm.

"I know that you are teaching him well," went on the boy's father. "Any life is better than this existence."

No, insisted the caseworker. We could not keep the child at the Center. Then the father suggested that we put the handicapped boy into an orphanage when he had completed his prosthetic training.

"Perhaps he will be adopted," he said.

Too many of the children in Korean institutions have parents who are unable or who do not wish to support them. We could not blame this father for allowing others to assume the care of his son, yet we felt that the child belonged in his own home with his own family. The social worker decided to refer the case to another agency, which might accept it on the basis of foster home care. If the boy could receive the same amount of support money which would be paid to an orphanage director, yet live in his own home, the whole family would be a little better off.

During the years of recovery which have followed the Korean War, the Korean people have begun to assume responsibility for their own problems. They are still dependent upon foreign aid to some extent, but they are showing eagerness and determination to manage their own affairs. This includes a real effort of government to cooperate with voluntary agencies in areas of public health and education. Progress has been made in the treatment and prevention of leprosy and tuberculosis, in vocational training, family planning, and social services. But in spite of a better standard of living and advances in medicine which should keep more parents alive longer, there seem to be more children in Korean orphanages than there ever were before. Korean social workers who have made surveys of the orphan problem tell us that the majority of these orphanages depend upon foreign support. Their report disclosed that a large percentage of the children who are fed, clothed, and educated in the orphanages are not really orphans at all. Like the little amputee boy who came to our Center, they have at least one living relative, and many of them have families living close-by the orphanage.

The question which immediately arises is why such children are in the orphanage. Anyone with an elementary acquaintance in psychology knows how institutional life can damage a child emotionally, and Korea is full of the proof of such damage. One such disturbed child was a patient at the amputee center. He and his brother had been raised in the orphanage, even though their grandmother lived in her own house nearby. The children visited her often and spent holidays and special days with her. A deep bitterness colored the sixteen-year-old boy's whole view of life. He felt that he had been cast off by his family. He was ashamed to call the orphanage "home."

Anyone with some understanding of the value which Korean culture places upon family and clan can appreciate this boy's feelings. And anyone who has met parents who struggle with such poverty that their little ones live on the edge of starvation can understand their reasons for putting the children into an orphanage. The relatives know where the little ones are; they know that they will be fed and clothed. They hope that with foreign support the children will also receive an education. The family is able to claim relationship to the child at any time it becomes convenient.

The appeal of a child is universal, and orphan sponsorship is a favorite charity for foreigners. Children are wonderful publicity gimmicks and, unfortunately, they are sometimes used that way. But in Korea, as everywhere else, the child is a dependent part of the family. It is the parent who usually needs the help. Although the word "orphan" is almost a magical formula in America, in a country which places such stress upon blood lines and family trees, it is a disgrace which a child is forced to carry with him all his life. Perhaps conditions have improved by this time, but I remember the day that one of our house servants lied to us about his parents. He was afraid that if he admitted that he had grown up in an orphanage, we would assume that no one had ever taken the time to teach him the proper way to live.

The most pathetic orphans are those who realize that they are dependent upon public charity. To visit an orphanage and to watch impressionable little children who have been taught to sing and perform for the benevolent guest makes one wonder how many of Korea's professional beggars received their first training in this way.

Recognizing the welfare of the child himself, voluntary agencies in Korea are seeking to support orphans and "pseudo-orphans" by foster care. They encourage destitute parents to keep their families together by giving them monthly support for the children. They encourage childless families to take in orphaned children and give them a home. In this way, the Korean people showing their willingness to accept responsibility with the cooperation of the foreign people, progress is being made in dealing with the orphan problem in Korea.

Once before we had been able to help a family through foster care. A pregnant woman who had lost an arm became widowed and was faced with the task of supporting two other children. At first she managed to keep herself and her little ones alive by selling candy—earning about twenty cents a day. But with the progression of pregnancy, she was unable to endure the long hours of walking. When she came to be fitted for a new arm, she told the social worker of her predicament. She was worried about the crisis which the impending birth would bring to her family.

The mother made no appeal. She seemed to have a sound sense of business and a strong desire to keep her family together. Somehow she would carry on—if only she could find a solution that would tide them over the few days when she would be unable to work at all. She was referred to Foster Parent Plan. The cooperation between the seventy-one organizations which made up the Korea Association of Voluntary Agencies and the close working relationship between missionaries of different denominations, between Catholics and Protestants, was one of the greatest blessings that we experienced. All worked for a common goal, and although opinions and methods sometimes differed, there was mutual respect and assistance.

Not every case which applied for admission at the rehabilitation center was accepted. Some were denied service because their physical condition obviously would not tolerate an active rehabilitation program. As news of our opening spread throughout the country, many old cases sought readmittance. Their limbs were checked and repaired; they were interviewed by the Korean social workers who were interested in finding out the reasons why they had come back. In many cases it was plain to us that we had failed in the past to meet the specific needs of the handicapped people.

Seldom was a patient turned away because of his age. One of the most delightful cases was a seventy-seven-year-old grandmother who had hobbled in with a cane to politely request repairs on her artificial leg. The leg was an eight-year-old below-knee model, wired and tied together in several places. The old woman was having difficulty in walking because of an ankle bolt which had worn through and poked against her stump.

The white head bobbed knowingly when we pointed this out in clinic. "Too old," she stated, matter-of-factly.

"Why didn't you have it fixed before?" asked our limb maker, as he picked away at the bits of string and wire which held the leg. Grandmother bared her remaining teeth in a cheerful grin.

"Too old," she repeated. "I, myself—too old."

She explained how her relatives had jeered at her desire for a new leg. A woman who is ready for the grave has no need of such fancy attachments. So she had simply walked off one day to find the Center by herself. The spunky little old amputee was given a new leg, and she practiced her walking until she was satisfied that she could walk home with pride. Such determination gave us all hope and enthusiasm. The new Center seemed to be off to a wonderful start.

13

Life anywhere is easier and more fun if it is seasoned with humor. Korea is no exception. We could giggle anonymously the day the lights went out in an auditorium and we fumbled into the wrong rest room; we even thought it was rather neat when a thief managed to tiptoe between the bodies of four children, who were sleeping on the floor, to get a television set out of a third story window. And everyone but Joy laughed when her beloved cat brought a live mouse into bed with her and began to toss it around and tease it. But it was hard to find anything to laugh about during the annual rainy season. At first, when the hot and humid air became too oppressive, we welcomed the rain. The whole landscape was washed clean and the familiar scenes were softened by the fresh mist.

Once it had started, the rain could not stop. Roads turned into sticky bogs or just washed away altogether. Everyone who walked outside was splashed by the red mud. We could wash the clothes, but we could not get them dry. The mold began to grow on books in the library and over the shoes that stood in the closet. Sometimes big patches of mildew appeared on the wallpaper which peeled from the damp cement walls. Rivers rose ominously higher and higher until at last, fed by torrents of muddy water which rushed down the mountainsides, they spilled over completely to cover nearby villages and carry away everything in their path.

Even though the rains came regularly every July, we did not have sense enough to prepare for them. One year we even started off to the beach on vacation the day that the rainy season started. Three families in three Land Rovers began the seventy-mile trek on a sunny morning, with the truck containing the provisions trailing behind. We had progressed only a few miles when the rain began, lightly at first. Soon the rivulets had become boiling waterfalls, tumbling down into the ditches alongside the road and often covering the entire roadway. A Land Rover is a hardy vehicle and can grind its way through almost anything, but thirteen miles from the end of our journey we met a bridge that had washed out. There was simply no way to get across the river, so we had to turn back and make a wide detour. The whole trip took seventy-two hours.

One year we had to move from one house to another on the first of July. There is no moving van in Korea, so our possessions were piled on the back of a truck. The mattresses were wet and mud-stained; then the electricity in the new house was shut off for three days, so we had no way to dry them out. Worse, the contents of the freezer began to thaw. Everyone else was in some kind of trouble too, so there was no help for it. We had moved into a beautiful new house, only to discover that the workman who laid the bricks in the chimney had tried to save concrete by using more sand. Since the roof was flat, the water soon washed out the sandy mortar between the chimney bricks and came cascading down the fireplace into the living room. As the wallpaper loosened from the walls, the ceiling tiles began to swell and drip, and the wall paneling warped before our eyes, I watched in frustration. Day after day we mopped, and day after day it rained.

Just as we were sitting down to supper one evening, Joy looked out the front windows. She called our attention to a tiny boy who stood weeping piteously at the end of our driveway. Passersby stared at him as he shivered in the cold rain and then they walked on. After half an hour we could stand no more of it and prevailed upon Mr. Kim to bring the child inside. Kim was uncertain. In Korea, people do not go about meddling in other people's affairs. But he put on his raincoat and splashed out barefooted to carry the little fellow back with him into the house. Mary and Joy were delighted. They dried the child and comforted him and dressed him in their outgrown clothing. He seemed to enjoy the attention, and allowed himself to be fed and petted.

"Can we adopt him, Dad?" asked Mary.

Mr. Kim explained to her that the baby must have a mother somewhere, but the girls were sure that the child had been abandoned in our driveway so that we could take him in. This made John uneasy. He did not want to keep the little boy overnight, but to put him back out in the rain was unthinkable. Then he had an idea.

"Put him in the car," he said. "I'll take him to the amputee center and let the social workers handle it. We'll stop at the police station and tell the police that he is there in case his parents are looking for him."

So they drove off—Father guiding the sturdy Rover with practiced proficiency through the deep, watery ruts and motherly little Mary sitting beside him with the Korean child on her lap. In the back of the Rover sat a dubious Mr. Kim who would serve as interpreter. I followed them from the window as they zig-zagged down the churned-up road and when the car was out of sight I watched the villagers go about their business, seemingly oblivious of the rain.

Then I noticed a young woman with an infant tied to her back and a full market basket on her head. A thought occurred to me. Perhaps she was the little boy's mother. When she had walked off to the market he had followed her part way and given up when she pulled too far ahead. He could simply have stood there, waiting for her to return as he cried in the rain.

The woman walked down the path and disappeared into one of the village houses. She emerged very quickly and darted into her neighbor's house. Running from one house to another, she appeared distracted and I became more and more convinced that my hunch was correct. As the young mother began walking up the path behind her house up the mountain, I began to walk to the nearest house in the village.

In broken Korean I managed to convey the message that we had a Korean child at our house. The news traveled so fast through the village that I had not gone a hundred yards toward home before the mother was running behind me.

She was followed by her husband, who spoke English. They accepted the explanation of why we had brought the baby to the

Center and we all sat down to wait for John's return. It was a long wait, and I suspected that the anxious parents began to think that the boy had been kidnapped after all. We talked, the father and I, and finally the mother left us to go back to the new baby. I learned that the young man was employed at the U.S. Army library. He was a college graduate and it was pleasant to visit with him. But where was my husband?

After dropping Mary and the child off at the amputee center, John and Mr. Kim had gone to the police station. While Kim explained the mission, John stopped in at his favorite barber shop and while the girl barber solicitously shaved him, massaged his neck muscles, and cleaned out his ears and nostrils, I was trying to reassure a polite, but impatient father. When at last we saw the Rover bucking its way back through the mud it was already dark. Poor John had to turn it around and take it right back through the ruts.

Our new house was built on the slope of a hill, overlooking a pleasant valley. Behind us, small green pines and thick acacia trees covered the incline and sheltered song birds and pheasants. In front of us, the ground declined to a plain, then rolled away again to form hills against the skyline. From the study window I could watch people working in the fields and moving through the villages below us. Sometimes there would be a group of women, squatting with wide-spread knees—skirts tucked under them, heads tied up in white towels. Beside them, on the ground, were the little round baskets in which they gathered the greens they were digging. As I watched this activity, I could not help but envy the little old ladies as they bent easily from their waists to the ground to pull up the greens—this was a toe-touching exercise that left me aching at half their age!

In the spring the hills became lovely with the lavenders of wild azalea against the green. Here and there, the big gray rocks broke out in craggy relief or the pattern was broken by the bulge of a grave mound. I lived in the house long enough to see a big bulldozer climbing my hills and making big gashes in their sides for a new housing project. Already man-made rockwalls were beginning to crawl around the side of the hill. High on the top a bare spot showed where squatters had cut down the trees to build their huts. Before long the hill would be full of shacks and where the trees have been cut down the ground will become eroded. The whole beautiful picture will become another eyesore. This is the way it has gone in Korea.

To the right of the house the road cut through a pass in the mountain, and beyond the pass one could see more hills, mauve colored in the sunshine or gray in the morning mists. Beyond these hills the halcyon skies, which are the joy of every Korean, softened all the colors and blended them together. The Korean student never fails to remind us of the unusually beautiful azure sky when he writes a letter. In a country where there is so much that is ugly, I find that touching.

Sloping down out of the pass and past our house, the road carried with it the mainstream of Korean life. I watched a nun, walking past rapidly with long, determined strides. Her face was hidden by her habit, but she must have been Korean even though she had the stride of an American. All day long this road was filled with schoolchildren—tiny ones, walking to and from their classes. School in Korea is held in shifts and the children have about two hours of class each day, including Saturdays. For this they trudge miles in all kinds of weather with their schoolbags on their backs. When it rained they dawdled in the puddles, their bright plastic umbrellas making little pools of color above their heads. Those ingenious umbrellas, made on light bamboo struts, are called "one-day umbrellas" and cost only ten cents each. The children walked in segregated groups . . . first a knot of boys, then the girls, hugging each other in groups of two or three. The schools are not coeducational, so the boys and girls might not even know each other. They looked so small from the window that I often wondered how they would find their way home again.

Once I saw a crowd of teen-age boys, walking together on the hill road. Suddenly one of them threw himself flat in the middle of the gravel highway. One by one, the others followed his example. I was fascinated by the strange behavior. Down the hill behind them, the driver of a coal truck was forced to slow his vehicle in order to avoid running over the prone bodies in the road. As the truck slowed to a stop, the lads on either end jumped to their feet and ran behind it. They quickly tossed coal briquettes from the load on the truck into sacks which they carried. By the time the driver and his assistant realized what was going on, four bags had been filled and carried off into the ditch. Half a dozen boys were still in the road, but the two men on the truck must have figured that the coal probably wouldn't be weighed anyhow. They climbed back into the cab of their vehicle and drove on.

I felt like God—sitting up there in the big house looking down over the long road and the two villages. I had an overall view of Korean life. But unlike God, I had no control over the drama which unfolded before me.

❦ 14

E veryone who has read the Bible has felt a compassion for the leper. Leprosy was a stigma; the leper was an outcast. He was not allowed to live inside the camp or within the city walls. Wherever he passed, he had to announce his loathesome presence by the shout, "Unclean! Unclean!" It was impossible to conceal the disease for long because of the havoc it effected on the person's face and extremities. The clawlike hands and the distorted features were repulsive; amputations of the fingers and toes soon made the victim useless and reduced him to begging. Quite naturally, people in Bible times believed that leprosy was a special curse sent by God.

Authorities today generally are agreed that the disease we call "leprosy" is not the same disease spoken of in the Bible. Although it has many of the same characteristics, it is dissimilar in many ways. The common term in use for the infectious disease which is prevalent in so many Eastern lands today is "Hansen's disease." It is characterized by such symptoms as the loss of facial hair, partial or total facial paralysis, absorption of certain tissues in nose, fingers, and toes, and complete loss of sensation in some of the afflicted areas of the body. Although the attitude of society in some places has been changed by public education, the victims of this disease, still known as "lepers," are feared and segregated in most of those countries where the disease is common.

The population of Korea includes more than one hundred thousand leprosy patients. Many registered lepers live in segregated colonies or in leprosariums. Although some of the mission groups have provided hospital or clinical treatment for them, the general public is afraid of anyone who shows the symptoms of Hansen's disease and at the first visible sign of the disease casts him out. Even after the malady has run its course, the sight of the distorted features and limbs is too gruesome and the lepers are unwelcome in normal society. So the cured patients band together in little colonies, doomed to a miserable and lonely existence until they die.

The Korean government became concerned about the plight of its leprosy-afflicted citizens after all leprosy agencies made a united effort to cooperate in controlling the disease. The Church World Service Rehabilitation Center was invited to join this cooperating committee. Our concern for the leprosy patients began with the few who appeared at the Center with amputations. Further investigation revealed about a thousand Koreans who had suffered major amputations because of leprosy.

With a special grant from the Mission to Lepers of New Zealand, a pilot project was established at one of the leprosy clinics. At first our aim was to develop special prosthetic devices which would meet the particular needs of the cases there. Many of the amputations had been caused by poor medical care and treatment. Some of them had resulted from ignorance. This was especially true of many of the cases in the leprosariums. Injury or infection which the patient had not even noticed in the anesthesized limb was the beginning of serious trouble.

According to one report which came from a government-run leprosarium, the patients used to perform amputations on one another. The report took note of the fact that prejudice on the part of the public resulted in a loss of will in the patients. They had no desire to become self-sufficient outside the leprosarium, and some had been there as long as forty years.

In India and in Africa specialists in leprosy had developed various types of corrective shoes to relieve or prevent the large, infectious ulcers which form on the soles of the feet of the leprosy patients. We began to work on a special footwear for the Korean cases, in the hope that amputations could be prevented. Taking the standard Korean man's rubber shoe, we thickened the sole with a layer of cellulose. The shoe still looked like any other man's shoe, but it protected the bottom of the foot from the sharp stones and rough paths that are unavoidable in Korea.

The pilot project was set up at the Southern Presbyterian leper colony in Soonchun, on the southern coast of Korea, under the supervision of Dr. Stanley Topple. Two competent prosthetic technicians from the rehabilitation center staff were sent to the Soonchun colony to train patients there in the skill of making artificial limbs. Many of the Korean leprosy amputees were wearing crude, homemade, poorly-fitted prostheses, and some had damaged their stumps so badly that they would need surgery before they could be fitted with artificial limbs.

As interest in the project grew, several doctors expressed a desire to cooperate. The American Leprosy Mission offered a sizable grant to enable our limb maker to go abroad to study the latest techniques in prosthetics for leprosy patients. We chose Hong Kong for his training, rather than to follow the popular pattern of sending him to the United States. The ideas which have been successful and which receive so much publicity in Western countries often are not practical in the Orient, or they may be too expensive for a developing country to maintain. There is a real need for the exchange of ideas among professional workers in Asian countries and also a need to develop centers in Asia where they can go to train in special skills. The limb maker's course in Hong Kong was a step in this direction.

Our primary task was not to manufacture limbs. The limb shop was only a part of the rehabilitation center. It is senseless to build an expensive limb for a leprosy patient, to expect him to spend a great deal of effort in learning to use it well, and then to keep him in a colony where all his needs receive attention without any effort on his part. Our interest was in returning these patients to productive living—to break down the prejudice of those who had no contact with leprosy, to remove their fears of the disease. And in this we had to begin with the workers in the amputee rehabilitation center.

There was consternation when John suggested taking arrested

cases of leprosy as inpatients. The staff members protested that not one person would remain in the dormitories. Acceptance does not come by force, so John compromised—the amputees who had leprosy would live in a rooming house in the city, would eat their meals outside, but would appear in clinic with other patients. Perhaps more was gained than lost by this compromise. Instead of moving from one institutionalized setup into another, the amputee lepers lived in the community. They ate in public eating places and they used public conveyances to travel back and forth to the Center. It was a breakthrough.

The first leprosy case to be fitted with prosthesis at the Seoul rehabilitation center was Mr. Min. His disease had been diagnosed when he was twenty years old and he had spent five years living in a leprosarium. During this time his parents died and his family was scattered. While the young man was being fitted with his new leg and learning to walk on it, the social worker found an elder brother of the patient living in a small southern town. In spite of violent opposition from the brother's wife, he succeeded in enlisting the cooperation of this brother and of the community leaders to resettle Mr. Min among them. Mr. Min had received some training in barbering and in chicken raising, so the amputee center agreed to provide him with a set of barber tools if he could pass the government examination for the barber's license.

A second patient who came in at about the same time was Mr. Yoon. He had also suffered from active leprosy for five years and had lost one leg by amputation. His left fingers were mutilated, and his face had been disfigured by the disease. With the cooperation of the local government officials in the community where the patient's elderly mother was living, he was helped to rehabilitate himself. When his sisters, who had refused to associate with him during the two years that he lived in the leprosy colony, heard that the community had accepted him again, they also offered their help. Mr. Yoon and his sisters have started a fish-selling shop, and follow-up investigation by the social worker indicated that the man had successfully been weaned from sheltered living.

Some other cases were more depressing. One man had lived in the leprosy colony since he was a child, but his disease had been declared negative seven years before he came to the rehabilitation center. He had removed his own name from the list of government citizens in an attempt to end his existence socially and legally. But he hated the life in the colony and left it to beg. Since there was no way to establish the fact that he was still a Korean citizen, it was difficult to secure the cooperation of a community to receive him.

Another resident of the leprosarium had been there six years and was resigned to the fact that his relations with normal people were completely severed. He steadfastly refused all offers of help. The social worker would not give up; gradually the man gained hope, and finally he presented himself at the Center for rehabilitation. With him he brought an oil painting of the crucifixion which he had made with his own clawed fingers.

Kim Young Hyuk was intensely interested in this aspect of rehabilitation. He felt that if only one or two leprosy cases could be fully rehabilitated and followed up, we would make more progress than if we could show impressive statistics of patients who had been fitted with limbs but who eventually returned to the isolation of the colony. Mr. Kim realized that the rehabilitation of leprosy patients involved more than a physical rehabilitation. Their social, vocational, and psychological needs would call for the best efforts of many skilled people for many years. He believed that those who once left the shelter of the leprosarium should never return as long as their disease remained arrested.

During his ministry on earth, Christ healed lepers. He did not fear them or run from them. "Those who are well," he said, "do not need a physician, but those who are sick." This included that despised group who were afflicted with leprosy. Christ had compassion on them.

The church of Christ, following his example, has pioneered in the medical treatment of the leper. Missionaries in all lands have set an example which is slowly being followed by enlightened governments. Although no missionary has been given the power of the Lord to heal the sick with a word, many have demonstrated the divine love and compassion of the Savior by bringing relief and restoration through modern medical means and dedicated service.

They have tried to educate the patient, his family, and the society in which he lives so that his disease may be better understood and less feared. Missionary doctors can restore the use of his hands to a crippled victim of leprosy now; they can remove the visible evidence of his disease by rebuilding his nose or ears or transplanting scalp hair to form new eyebrows; they can prevent blindness by ingenious operations on paralyzed eyelids. Christian doctors and rehabilitation workers can also restore to the disfigured leprosy patient a new sense of personal dignity by teaching him that his soul is free. The genuine concern and self-sacrificing love which has been demonstrated to the patients at the Christian hospitals in Korea and elsewhere is a real witness to the mercy and love of Jesus Christ. The body is treated but the soul is not neglected. Many a leper has heard the Lord say to him, "Thy sins are forgiven," and he has gone out to spread the news to his fellow sufferers.

15

The day that we received the news of Kim Ki Sun's adoption was a glad day at the Center. The little boy had been living in the home of Mrs. Song for two years, and although the Songs treated him as if he were one of their own children, the boy knew that he was not. We knew that, although the Songs never complained, the presence of the lively, aggressive outsider must often be unsettling in their home. Both Mr. and Mrs. Song were leg amputees and they were very helpful in teaching Kim Ki Sun to care for his stump and his artificial leg. But they were gentle people and Kim was a bundle of energy. The four Song children were well-disciplined, extremely polite, and restrained in public. Little Kim tried to imitate them but he was irrepressible and often had to be admonished by the mild-mannered Deacon Song. His artificial leg did not limit his activity at all, and his wild background as a beggar boy was often an embarrassment in his foster home.

To prepare him as much as possible for the tremendous change in his life, Kim Ki Sun came to live with us. Before the arrival of his new parents from California, we would give him a "crash course" in Americanization. We tried to teach him enough English words so that he could communicate just a little and establish a relationship with his parents. They had decided to keep two syllables of his name, perhaps in the mistaken notion that the last syllable was his Korean surname. But being addressed as "Kim" or "Kimgi" was a minor change for the ten-year-old boy. He was put into a room by himself and for the first time in his life he began to sleep in a bed. He was expected to keep the toilet flushed and clean. He learned to eat strange foods with a fork instead of his chopsticks. Worst of all, he had to go to bed at nine o'clock in the evening. Kimgi, who was used to retiring when it became dark and rising when it became light, found American habits exceedingly strange.

He was puzzled by our reaction of horror and dislike when he swung the kittens by their tails. Mary and Joy found this hard to forgive, although we tried to explain to them that Kimgi's early learning had not included kindness to animals. Dirk was annoyed by Kimgi's curiosity—he poked into everything and managed to damage some of Dirk's cherished possessions. John and I were often distressed by his easy lies. Kimgi was an exceptionally bright child and full of ideas. He was eager to help and sometimes in his attempt to "fix" things he broke them beyond repair. This made Mr. Kim nervous and he would scold the little boy.

The adjustment must have been even harder for Kimgi than it was for us, although he did his best to cooperate with our strange ways. When he could stand it no longer, he simply walked out. This threw us into a panic. We knew that Kimgi had once been a beggar boy and that with no trouble at all he could lose himself among the beggar horde again. How could we possibly explain that to his new parents?

Mr. Kim dashed down the road Kimgi had taken. Where he found him or what was said between them, they did not tell us. Mr. Kim explained that Kimgi had decided he did not want to go to America after all. We were sorry about being the cause of the boy's unhappiness. It is not easy for a child of ten to adapt himself to an entirely new way of life. Kimgi was an independent and intelligent boy, or we would never have attempted to change his entire environment at that age. In spite of the uncertainty and discomfort the change would cause him, we were convinced that it was the right course of action. In America, the amputation of one leg would never hinder him—whereas to an orphan in Korea it could be a heavy handicap.

Mrs. Song came to our rescue. When she heard of the difficulties Kimgi and we were having, she came to visit him. She told him that we realized that he could not learn our strange ways in a few weeks and we were not angry at his mistakes. Perhaps, she suggested, when he became discouraged or lonely in the big American house, he might like to run down to the Center and visit there. Kimgi seized upon the escape and became a frequent visitor at the rehabilitation center. He was received as a celebrity—a boy who had attained the dream of going to U.S.A. The Korean people made much of him, and Kimgi enjoyed his privileged position.

When he had found this vent for his energies, Kimgi became more relaxed at the house. He no longer felt like a prisoner. We also relaxed, knowing that if we missed him he was playing at the Center. One day, when both Mr. Kim and Kimgi had gone out, I was interrupted by a pounding at the door. A peek out of the window told me that the caller was only a beggar. Long before, we had adopted the policy that we did not give money or clothing to beggars at the door. Mr. Kim's orders were firm. "Give them bread, if they are hungry," we had told him. "They cannot sell the bread as they will the rice, and if they are not hungry enough to eat it it will only spoil."

The ragged, dirty old man pounded on my door with his stick. "Beggar! Beggar!" he called out.

I handed him two biscuits through the half-open door, but this only made him angry. He threw the bread down on the cement step and spit on it. So I shut the door and went back to my typewriter. Although I was unaware of it, the side door of the house had remained unlatched when Kimgi had used it to exit. The old man found it open and walked through it into the hallway, calling loudly for money.

Frightened and angry, but determined not to give him any money, I tried to chase him back down the hall with a broom. "Get out!" I was shouting, almost hysterically, when Kimgi appeared in the doorway behind the beggar. He took in the situation at once and assumed command. Speaking very deferentially to the old man, he walked quietly with him through the door outside. I could see him, crouching alongside the beggar at the roadside, talking earnestly.

When Mr. Kim returned, I prodded him to ask Kimgi what he and the old beggar had talked about. The child began a long, animated story. It was evident that he had enjoyed his conversation. Mr. Kim interrupted occasionally to translate parts of the story for me—Kimgi had been reliving his own begging days, asking the man about old friends and acquaintances "on the road." Although he had lived only ten years, Kimgi had crowded a great deal of colorful experience into them.

The new parents were arriving with a planeload of eighty people on a chartered Flying Tiger plane. Most of the passengers had brought sleeping bags and intended to camp out in the chapel at the Holt orphanage farm. But we had invited Kimgi's parents to stay at our home in order that they might have more opportunity to get to know their son and so that they could spend some time at the Center learning about his artificial leg and how to care for it.

At midnight, one Sunday, the plane arrived. We had been waiting at the airport since eight, but we were not as tired as the people who rushed off the plane. Kimgi was overwhelmed by hugs and kisses from his weary parents and although he appeared bewildered by their show of love for him, he enjoyed it. It was two o'clock by the time we reached our home, and we were feeling very sorry for all those others who had flown so far and now had to endure the tedious, rutted ride out to the Holt farm. Before going to bed, our guests presented their son with their arrival gifts. First there was the wristwatch and the new clothes . . . then the viewmaster and the camera. At home, Kimgi, there is a pony and a bicycle and there are two sisters waiting for you. Kimgi was impressed by the sudden wealth, but the abundance of love which was given with it had more effect on him. Embarrassed and made shy at first by the kissing and hugging, he finally accepted the fact that these people loved him and were going to be a real mother and father for him at last. He began to respond to their affection with kisses of his own, and he stayed close to them. When we talked to him, he did not hear us. He ignored any orders given by Mr. Kim, and began to give orders to Mr. Kim instead. Our home was his home, and as such he freely offered it to his "mamma" and "dad." Nothing was too good for Kimgi's mamma. Mr. Kim good-naturedly submitted to Kimgi's demands and shared in the happiness of the new family.

A script writer and a photographer from Hollywood had come along with the plane to do a documentary film on the mass adoption. They decided to include the story of the amputee orphan, and so we entertained them at the Center and in our home. Since our guests were eager to visit the Holt farm and to greet their fellow travelers, we made the long drive out to the farm one day. On the way back to the city, the film-makers inquired about Mr. Holt and his work with the orphans. "What do you think of it?" one asked.

I replied that I was worried. "It is a one-man operation," I said, "and Mr. Holt is not a well man. He might drop dead anytime . . . today or tomorrow or next week . . ."

We traveled leisurely, stopping often to photograph the children alongside the road as they dug up the green shoots to put in the family food pots. The guests were shocked by the sight of three- and four-year-old tots with their little round baskets and huge, pointed knives. We admired the picturesque flat-topped Korean pine trees, bent and knarled and beautiful, tipped to one side by many winds. We took note of the graceful swinging hips of the women ahead of us as they walked down the road carrying tubs full of produce on their heads.

There was much to delight the eyes of a photographer. The film captured a placid, fat granny waddling in her little rubber shoes down the path between the rice paddies and the pot-bellied male child who was making use of the most convenient facilities to relieve himself. We paused in the village where it was market day and we went exploring through the crowds. Old crones, sitting in their sunny doorways picking lice out of the children's hair, took little notice of us; but the children who played naked in the muddy water of the ditches or ran about catching dragonflies in their home-made nets left their play to follow at our heels. They were curious about the Korean boy with the American adults, but Kimgi disdained them. He had suddenly become an American and the son of Americans. "Git!" he shouted rudely at the children in Korean language, and he ignored their efforts to speak to him.

When the Rover arrived at the Center, an urgent message awaited. Mr. Holt had died suddenly while we were on the road back to Seoul. Would the two film-makers return as quickly as possible?

The Holt office in Seoul had no vehicle available, so our driver turned around and headed back to the farm in order that tragedy might be documented. The eighty parents and their newly-adopted Korean children said a final good-bye to Harry Holt before he was buried in the mud of his farm. Slogging through the mire to his gravesite and mingling their tears with the rain that fell throughout the service, they buried him in the country to which he had given everything he had to give.

The Flying Tiger departed from Kimpo airport amid chaos. We spent the entire afternoon at the airport and again found legitimate use for our carefully-hoarded supply of tranquilizer pills. At last all the tense parents and all the tired children had been herded into the plane and we saw Kimgi on his way to America. It had been a hectic week.

Between trying to be everybody's friend, we occasionally dropped in at the amputee center to catch up on our business there. The tours went on as usual—one for six women on a round-the-world trip, another for the Protestant Women of the Chapel, and another which included about seventy-five American soldiers on retreat. There were VIP's and tourists who were brought by their missionary friends. The staff members were very gracious about the interruptions and the patients had become accustomed to visitors and showed no embarrassment. They answered questions freely and offered to show off their quarters or their accomplishments. Some of the visitors were pastors, teachers, leaders who are influential in their home churches. But most of them were American soldiers who came from the servicemen's centers run by the National Council of Churches or the Lutheran denominations. We realized that mission activity is not a part of the experience of most Christian young people in America, and when a young GI comes into contact with this mission outreach he sees his church in action overseas. Most of the GIs see very little of the Korean country, and of what has been done to improve conditions in Korea. Usually, when they return to America, they speak of Korea and of their Army tour there with bitterness and contempt. We considered it good public relations to interrupt our work with these tours for them. Through a single GI who returns to his home church in America and tells what he has seen in Korea, we probably could reach more people than we would by pictures and articles in church magazines which people nowadays have no time to read. In one month, 435 American soldiers passed through our Center.

Usually, as we guided them through the Center, we introduced them to some of the patients. "This six-year-old girl is dying of cancer . . . we cannot send her back to her home . . . This handsome little boy required four plastic operations before we could fit him with a leg. He had been so severely burned that he was bent almost double with scar tissue when his father first brought him in . . . and this friendly patient is the same man who choked on his meals the first few days that he ate in our dining room. He could not eat when he remembered that his family was starving . . . Here is an orphan, brought to us by a Methodist pastor. His stumps are so short that they are a problem to the arm maker. But see how he feeds himself with his foot! He is a good boy and bright enough, but he is too old now for primary education at the public school. What can we do with him?"

We explained to the visitors that the people whom they saw at the Center were only a small part of the case load which we handled there. Many were treated on an outpatient basis. But we had found that the fellowship of others, the sharing of needs and of abilities, the encouragement which comes with another's progress are important factors in restoring self-confidence. Mothers who have left their own little ones at home are comforted by the need of another child for mothering. A man with no legs is carried on the back of a man who has lost a hand. And so they help each other—and by helping each other they are helping themselves. They learn and they have taught us that "no man is an island." Given an opportunity to give of themselves, they have taken their first steps back to personal responsibility.

16

We had returned to Korea in 1962 on a three-year contract with Church World Service, but we stayed four years. It was time to go.

It was hard to explain to our Korean friends why we must leave. No, it was not homesickness. Korea had become our home. Yes, we were happy and content in Korea. No, we did not believe that there was no more work that we could do there. Korea is full of challenges still.

Our American friends did not understand either. "Why must you leave if you like it there?" they wrote to ask us. And I wrote back:

"The simple answer is that our contract has ended. We have been working here on a year's extension, in fact. John felt that he owed this to the newly-organized Center."

The plan of Church World Service, they say, is to move out of ongoing institutional work and to concentrate on emergency relief. The trend in Korea is for government and private Korean agencies to take over the charities which were initiated by the foreign agencies. Negotiations are in progress with Yonsei University Medical Center to absorb the amputee project.

John's intention was to set up a "pilot project" in rehabilitation and his hope was that by the time he left Korea the medical center would be ready to take it over. If Korea and the medical profession there had not yet reached a point where it felt the need or was able to support a program of physical medicine, then there seemed to be no point in continuing the work with foreign funds and foreign personnel. Perhaps we must face the fact that there are other more important demands in Korea than the plight of the disabled.

Kim Young Hyuk did not accept the fate of the project with such equanimity. During the six years that he had served as John's assistant, he had become convinced that his people *must* accept this responsibility and he has become dedicated to the concept of total rehabilitation. Already he sees that for Yonsei University Hospital to take over the extensive program which has been carried on from the small rehabilitation center is an impossibility at the present time. Our goal of a social outreach, combined with a religious, medical, and prosthetic organization had made the project known throughout all Korea. Patients who had been hiding away for years came out of their holes and found their way to the rehabilitation center to ask for treatment. But in their complete dedication to the cause of the handicapped, our staff members at the Center had overlooked the demands of politics and bureaucracy which are the price of belonging to a larger organization. In our zeal to pervade the Korean society with a responsibility for the cripple, we had not spent enough time educating the regents of Yonsei University and medical center or the ruling powers of Church World Service . . . people whose dedication and goals naturally differed from ours. Beset with its own problems of overexpansion, lack of adequate funds, political intrigues, internal strife, and labor difficulties, Yonsei University Medical Center seemed the least likely choice for the continuance of our program.

It gave Mr. Kim no comfort to know that we were, in spite of all this, committed to an affiliation with Yonsei University Medical Center. When we left Korea, Mr. Kim would be left with the problem. John had pointed the course and it was time for him to withdraw his direction. He could see the travail which was ahead for Mr. Kim and he was well aware of the fact that Kim Young Hyuk, although knowledgeable in social work and rehabilitation procedure, had no status with the Yonsei faculty without a doctor's degree. He also realized that Mr. Kim would have problems with the Church World Service staff. Although not one foreign staff member had been in Korea longer than two years and although not one of the staff had any concept of what physical medicine or rehabilitation implies, the decisions which would affect the future of the entire program would now be of their making. Mr. Kim, as a Korean national, would not enjoy the same privilege in the CWS office that John had enjoyed as an American representative of the organization. This is regrettable, but it was nonetheless very true.

Our hope as we prepared to leave our post, was that Church World Service and Severance Hospital (Yonsei Medical Center) would recognize the careful and broad training that Mr. Kim had acquired. Perhaps they already realized that the two Korean gentlemen, Kim Young Hyuk and Dr. Kim, the orthopedist, combined an insight into the physical and social problems of their people that no foreigner could ever match. Perhaps Church World Service would appreciate the delicate balance which existed when John was not there and would support the rehabilitation program in its agony as the Korean people tried to take it over and nurture its growth. The project is at a crucial stage. We can only pray. We have done all we could do. To remain in Korea longer would only weaken the program from the Korean point of view. John had complete confidence in his staff; he had given them responsibilities and he had delighted in their performance. He knows that they are competent and no longer need a foreign director.

As we look back over the eight years' work in Korea, we are tempted sometimes to wonder what we have actually accomplished. Only eternity will tell the whole story. Only God knows how many lives have been changed through the love and mercy of the Lord Jesus as it was shown to these amputees. We pray that this witness may continue through the dedicated efforts of the doctors and nurses, social workers, and other staff members who have learned that their Christianity must operate horizontally as well as vertically.

One of the amputee patients, an intelligent, sensitive gentleman of about forty years, states it very well. Mr. Chang lost both arms about thirteen years ago and since then he has been completely dependent upon others. When his friends heard tales of the missionary amputee who had come to Korea to help the limbless,

Mr. Chang was frankly skeptical. He was familiar with Christianity, since he had turned to it immediately after the trauma of his amputation. Seeking understanding, he had been given sympathy and pity. And so, disappointed and disillusioned with the church, he had withdrawn from it.

However, he had nothing to lose by coming to the Christian rehabilitation center. So he became an inpatient and was fitted with artificial arms. He seemed to enjoy the activities and the companionship at the Center and when it was time for him to leave, Mr. Chang made a speech in clinic.

He told us that he had come expecting very little. At first the clumsy appliances had been too much to bear, but he had kept trying because of the encouragement given by staff members who really seemed to care. And now, went on the earnest little man, his whole life was changed. From being completely dependent, he was able to help himself with his personal needs. He showed us a letter that he had written to his little daughter "by his own hand." He beamed with joy when he described how the amputees in the dormitories all helped each other. He himself was teaching an illiterate boy how to read and write.

"In this place," said Mr. Chang, "I have seen Christianity act." He told how he had carefully watched the relationship of the staff members to the patients and to one another. Never before had he realized that real love and concern for others was the fruit of the Christian faith.

Our experience is very much like Mr. Chang's. We have learned the blessing of serving others. We have felt the richness of being needed, of being able to contribute. We have seen "Christianity act." Wherever we go, whatever life holds for us in the future, this is the gift which we will take with us from Korea.

🌷 Postscript

The Director of the Korea Church World Service sent a letter to the Asia Secretary of the New York office of Church World Service in August of 1966, one month after John's departure from Korea. He expressed his delight at the manner in which the team of Kim Young Hyuk (the new Director at the rehabilitation center) and Dr. Kim (the orthopedist at Severance Hospital) were carrying on the work. In the letter he praised the excellent training of Mr. Kim and he credited John with the development of Kim's talents and with his devotion to the cause of rehabilitation "for it was he who inspired and led him in this work."

The Korea Church World Service director had observed the fine teamwork between the two Korean men who had been left in charge of the Center. Each recognized that the other had a particular contribution to make. Each respected the role of the other. Mr. Kim was eager to get every patient back as an independent member of society. Dr. Kim's concern was with the care and treatment of the amputated stump, the fit and function of the prostheses, and the ability of the patients to use their new appliances.

Kim Young Hyuk began his work with dedication. Although he was aware that Severance Hospital had already offered the post he temporarily occupied, as Director at the rehabilitation center, to another man who was then receiving special training in rehabilitation in New York City, this was not a problem to Mr. Kim.

"I am glad to learn that a Korean man has an interest in

rehabilitation to the point of studying it on his own," he wrote to us. "I hope that he will come home and serve the handicapped in his own country. I do not seek a high position for myself, although I did demand the directorship of the amputee center after you left Korea because it seemed to me that I was most qualified to continue the concept of total rehabilitation you and I shared. However, when there is another man with real qualification for the job, I am willing to step down."

Mr. Kim was especially worried about his ability to control the budget, but he humbly depended upon the accountants at the rehabilitation center and in the Church World Service office to watch over his expenditures and to warn him if he spent unwisely or too freely. When we began to receive hints from others that Kim was not administering the funds as carefully as John had done before him, we asked him about it. He replied: "I understand that it is the job of the Korea Church World Service accountants and of the American comptroller in the office to put the brakes on me if I go beyond the limitation. But I have fought the tendency in the main office to meddle with me overmuch. I welcome visits by the Americans in Korea Church World Service to inquire into any matter at the Center, but they should not try to become directors of the Center themselves. That is my job."

By the end of the year 1966, the handwriting had appeared on the wall. Kim Young Hyuk was convinced of his ability to direct the work of rehabilitation in Korea. He had worked hard as an understudy in order to prepare himself for the job. He refused to be distracted from his purpose and he was not willing to humble himself to those who knew nothing about rehabilitation of the disabled simply because he was Korean and they were American, even though he realized full well that they not only controlled all the funds for the program but were also empowered to direct the decisions as to its future. Nor was Mr. Kim willing to accept the proper "low posture" as far as his relationships to other Koreans were concerned. Some of them disdained him because he had no status. He had neither earned a doctorate nor had he studied in

America. Others had been in the employ of the amputee center longer than had Mr. Kim and deeply resented his elevation to the position of director of the program. These snubs and the petty jealousy and rancor had been evidenced from time to time during John's leadership, but the fact that John was a foreigner had helped keep them in check.

Perhaps Mr. Kim was unduly stubborn. He pursued his own way, working day and night toward his goals, heedless of those who sought to trip him up. He was determined to convince the Korean public of its duties toward the disabled. Toward this end he worked to put his little magazine, *Human Family*, on a firm financial basis. He drafted the help of staff members, amputee students, and interested friends to sell subscriptions and get others to cooperate.

"What a busy job the amputee center director has to do!" Kim Young Hyuk wrote in a letter to us at the end of 1966. "It simply drives me crazy, day by day. Work, work, and work. Rarely do I leave the Center before nine in the evening. And I always work all day on Saturday. Guests, mostly tourists from abroad, keep coming. Reports must be written to the main office, to supporters here and abroad. The patient load has reached a record high of thirty-seven this week. Writing articles for the monthly magazine, the *Korea Times*, and some local magazines requires more and more time and study. It all deprives me of much time with my family. My wife has become cynical, commenting that without Kim Young Hyuk the whole rehabilitation center would certainly fall apart!

"The Human Family Program is getting more and more social acceptance, though it brings in little income. The other day the *Han'guk Ilbo* (a Korean daily newspaper) carried a small editorial praising the initiative of the magazine and urging all the people to subscribe to it. The editorial termed it a most realistic approach to the problem of the physically handicapped in Korea. The editor-in-chief of the newspaper had called me and said that he himself read the magazine every month and he wanted some additional information on it."

Although Mr. Kim was gratified with the public recognition that the little magazine received, he gradually became more and more discouraged about his job. The future of the amputee center looked gloomy to him. "They seem to be satisfied with the way I am running the Amputee Center," he wrote, "but they refuse to discuss the important question of how the handicapped people in this country can best be served. I keep on working and working the best way I can. That is all I can do. I pray the Lord for the future, but I confess that I do not have a firm faith that He will carry us through. Please pray for me and for the other workers here."

Mr. Kim's gloom was well-founded. The more he pushed for the independence of the rehabilitation program, the more distrust he aroused among the administrators at the Yonsei Medical Center and in the Korea Church World Service. He realized that if the work of rehabilitation was going to survive in Korea it would have to be self-supporting and so he submitted a proposal to separate the limb shop from the social work department. He expressed his dislike of dependence upon foreign funds and his hope of interesting Korean society in the care of its own handicapped.

Since there were only two social workers to cover the entire 300-bed Severance Hospital, Severance could see no sense in keeping a staff of six social workers at the rehabilitation center, which had a capacity inpatient load of thirty-six people. Mr. Kim attempted to describe the outreach of his social work staff—among crippled children and leprosy patients and their families and in follow-up work and home visits, but his pleas fell upon deaf ears. When he was pressured to discharge the social workers at the rehabilitation center, he flatly refused. He was deeply disturbed because those who negotiated the incorporation of the Church World Service Rehabilitation Center by Yonsei Medical Center seemed to fail to realize the tremendous investment in the development and training of this social work team. Mr. Kim looked upon these workers as the future of the cause of rehabilitation in Korea. He could not see them disbanded without a struggle, even though he knew that to struggle would probably cost him his job.

On April 25, 1967, Kim Young Hyuk resigned as director of the rehabilitation center. He told us about it by letter:

> The long fight has come to an end. I am sorry to have to tell you that I can serve no longer, but hope you will under-

stand that I have done my best. As a product of the Amputee Center, I could not raise the hatchet to chop away the program bit by bit. When I confronted the Church World Service Director this morning, he accused me of ignoring his instruction to dissolve the team of social workers. I will be replaced in my position as Director of the Rehabilitation Center by the man who is now the Director of Material Aid Department of Church World Service. I wish him well.

I am filled with emotions which are difficult to express. I loved the amputee program and I am thankful for it. I pray that the Lord will see to it that it is able to continue. Although there is no confirmation of the fact, I have heard that Korea Church World Service will abolish all scholarships for amputee students and all vocational training programs. I do hope that is not true.

I wish that I could believe that my leaving would save the program. But I do not think so. Nevertheless, I have advised the KCWS Director to pay attention to Korean community leaders who can and should be won to back up rehabilitation in Korea. As for me, I shall continue to work into Korean society through the Human Family Program. The awareness of Korean society for the handicapped people and the support of Korean people for this program should eventually be achieved. Everyone recognizes this need, but few dare to do something for it. I hope to try, even if it will mean personal sacrifice. Your continued advice and prayer would be appreciated.

This was the last news we have had of the Korea Amputee Rehabilitation Center. When Mr. Kim left, those social workers who were not discharged with him resigned in protest. Three went to America for further study. One has died. Another has accepted a position as teacher in a Social Workers Training Institute. The young chaplain, who was discharged at this time also, accepted a scholarship for graduate study in an American seminary.

Whatever the future holds for the Yonsei Medical Center's Rehabilitation Department, we do not feel that our work has been in vain. The seed has been planted. A competent prosthetic team has been trained. Throughout Korea there are amputees who have taken their places as useful and productive members of society. Some of them are concerned about helping others to rehabilitate themselves. The Korean public has become aware of the problem and of the efforts which were made to overcome it.

The Human Family Program made progress for awhile, but it was not strong enough to make it on its own. Although influential leaders took interest in the project, Mr. Kim was not able to carry the whole burden of its support alone. We do not know how much interest in the program remains in Korea.

In the last analysis, the future of rehabilitation in Korea must depend upon the Korean people themselves. It depends upon Korean Christians and their concern for their fellowmen. It will reflect the witness of the Korean Christian Church and the influence of those missionaries who were sent to guide the church. Many people have shared in building a foundation of a rehabilitation program for the handicapped in Korea and God has used it as a means to bring Korean people, whether they are crippled or whole, to fuller knowledge of him and joy in his service. For many years this project was an expression of the love and concern of Christians throughout the world for their Korean neighbors. This is the legacy which will remain in Korea.